usually caught so late. . . . A thorough guide to the basics of how lung cancer develops, risk factors, diagnosis, treatment options, and living well with lung cancer. . . . Practical issues such as insurance and estate planning, hospice care, caregiver support, and other concerns are very well covered. . . . For patients and at-risk people, potentially lifesaving information. . . . Recommended."   —*Library Journal*

"This timely book provides a wealth of useful information to general readers concerned about their health and healthcare providers. . . . The authors decimate a series of popular cultural myths regarding lung cancer, including: 'If you smoke, the damage is done, so there's no point quitting' and 'If you're diagnosed with lung cancer, the situation is hopeless.' Thus, in addition to providing knowledge and support, this book also offers hope."
                                                                  —*Tampa Tribune*

Further prais

Lung Cancer

n-
w
ne
se,
kly

n-
he
to

N,
ty

r-
d
se

c.

d
n
h

),
n

is
e

l,
g

f

experience to this work giving valuable information to physicians, patients, and their families. The clarity of the presentation is one of its strengths, allowing the reader to gain the needed insight for various issues."

—LaSalle D. Leffall, Jr., M.D., F.A.C.S.,
Charles R. Drew Professor of Surgery, Howard University Hospital

"Individuals with the diagnosis of lung cancer or who are at high risk for developing this 'number one killer' can be overwhelmed and misinformed because the facts are not presented in a compassionate, intelligent manner. *Lung Cancer* provides the fundamentals for this disease in the caring manner of an all-encompassing support group. This unique reference text is must reading for those confronted with (or worried about) a lung cancer diagnosis in order to face this challenge head-on with facts rather than potentially misleading fairy tales."

—Harvey I. Pass, M.D., chief, Thoracic Oncology,
Karmanos Cancer Institute

"As an advocate for lung cancer awareness, and as a survivor, it is refreshing to read such a comprehensive and lucid description of the disease, its treatments, and the various psychosocial tools available to help patients and caregivers. This book acts as a guide and inspiration in the management and care of lung cancer. A must read for those at risk for or diagnosed with lung cancer!"

—James Asher, executive director,
Alliance for Lung Cancer Advocacy, Support and Education

"Henschke, McCarthy, and Wernick are offering lung cancer diagnostees another way of looking at themselves and their environments. This is a good idea."   —Nikki Giovanni, poet and lung cancer survivor

"A comprehensive, vitally important book that can save thousands of lives in educating people for early detection and treatment of this killer disease. You can live after lung cancer, and here's how."

—Priscilla Dewey Houghton, playwright and lung cancer survivor

"As a person whose family was hit by this horrible disease, I wish this book was available four years ago. It answered every question that we needed to know."   —Susan Levine, patient advocate

"Henschke has made news with her investigations into the early detection of lung cancer—important because the disease is so lethal precisely because it is

LUNG CANCER

Myths, Facts, Choices – and Hope

Claudia I. Henschke, Ph.D., M.D.
and
Peggy McCarthy

with Sarah Wernick

 W. W. Norton & Company   New York • London

For information about permission to reproduce selections from this book, write to
Permissions, W. W. Norton & Company, Inc., 500 Fifth Avenue, New York, NY 10110

Manufacturing by The Courier Companies, Inc.
Book design by Joan Greenfield
Text drawings by Robin M. Jensen, Inner Visions

ISBN 0-393-04154-9
ISBN 0-393-32498-2 pbk.

W. W. Norton & Company, Inc., 500 Fifth Avenue, New York, N.Y. 10110
www.wwnorton.com

W. W. Norton & Company Ltd., Castle House, 75/76 Wells Street, London W1T 3QT

1 2 3 4 5 6 7 8 9 0

We dedicate this book to everyone affected by lung cancer and to those striving to help them. In our hearts are all who have died from this terrible disease, but who continue to inspire us.

CONTENTS

AN IMPORTANT MESSAGE FOR READERS

This book is not intended to offer you medical advice. Rather, we hope to improve your general understanding of lung cancer, so that you can communicate effectively with your doctors and nurses and make informed decisions about your treatment. There is no substitute for the care of qualified health care professionals who know your particular medical history and the details of your condition.

Though we've made every effort to ensure that the information we present is accurate and current, knowledge about lung cancer is advancing rapidly. Your medical team—your primary care physician, your oncology specialty physicians, and your oncology nurses—may have new information that can help you. Throughout the book we will urge you to speak with them about any questions or concerns, and to seek additional opinions if needed.

A Note about Telephone Numbers and Web Site Addresses

All telephone numbers and Web site addresses were rechecked for the paperback edition. Unfortunately, some of them may have changed since then.

If you can't reach a telephone number, check with Directory Assistance or an online telephone directory such as Switchboard (*http://www.switchboard .com*) or AnyWho (*http://www.anywho.com*). Or use the Web site address (if there is one) to find the current telephone number.

If a Web address doesn't work, try the following:

- Carefully retype the address. Even a minor mistake, like a single incorrect letter, can prevent you from reaching your online destination.

- Go to the Web site's home page and see if a menu or search box can lead you to the material you're looking for. The home page is the first part of the address, ending with *com*, *org*, or *gov*, before the first forward slash (/). For example, *http://www.lungcanceronline.org/therapy.htm* is a specific page on Lung Cancer Online; the home page is *http://www. lungcanceronline.org*.

- Use a search engine, such as Google (*http://www.google.com*) to look for the information elsewhere.

ACKNOWLEDGMENTS

This book would not have been possible without a great deal of assistance from many people. We would like to express our appreciation to all those who generously shared their expertise and offered us their support. We benefited greatly from their help. Of course, any remaining errors are our responsibility.

Throughout the book we describe many important advances against lung cancer. We are grateful to all the physicians and investigators who have contributed to these developments. A special thanks to the following medical colleagues who answered our queries and reviewed portions of the manuscript:

Paul Bunn, Jr., M.D., director of the University of Colorado Cancer Center in Denver, reviewed the chapter about chemotherapy and responded to many questions.

David Burns, M.D., of the School of Medicine at the University of California at San Diego, responded thoughtfully to our questions about smoking cessation and tobacco control; he also reviewed the chapters about lung cancer risk factors and smoking cessation.

Robert J. Ginsberg, M.D., of Toronto General Hospital in Canada, reviewed the chapter on surgery; in addition, he was a source of valuable advice and assistance early in the development of this book.

Frederic W. Grannis, Jr., M.D., of the City of Hope National Medical Center in Duarte, California, patiently responded to frequent questions on many subjects; he provided careful reviews of several chapters: the introductory chapters on lung anatomy and the development of cancer; diagnosis and staging; and surgery.

Michael Kalafer, M.D., FCCP, of the University of California at San Diego, generously made himself available to answer questions; he reviewed the chapters about lung anatomy and the development of cancer, as well as chapters about risk factors and diagnosis.

William Kostis, Ph.D., of Weill Medical College, helped assemble useful illustrative materials for the book.

Jim Mulshine, M.D., of the National Cancer Institute, contributed to the entire book with his thorough responses to our numerous questions; he also provided detailed comments on the chapters about lung cancer screening and diagnosis, chemotherapy, and clinical trials.

Harvey Pass, M.D., of Wayne State University in Detroit, Michigan, reviewed the chapter about surgical treatment of lung cancer, offering many important additions and clarifications; his patient replies to dozens of queries are reflected in many other chapters as well.

Julianna Pisch, M.D., of the Beth Israel Medical Center in New York, provided helpful comments on an early version of the chapter on radiation oncology.

Michael Smith, M.D., FACC, FACS, president of the Georgia Institute for Lung Cancer Research, carefully reviewed chapters about risk factors and diagnosis, as well as the chapter about surgery.

Charles Thomas, M.D., of the University of Texas Health Science Center in San Antonio, offered a painstaking review of our chapter on radiation therapy, with many very helpful specific suggestions for improving it.

Alvaro Vallejo, M.D., of Weill Medical College, read an early draft of the chapter about radiation therapy, patiently answered questions, and provided important clarifications.

Lou Wallace, M.Div., Th.M., of Hospice and Palliative Care of Greensboro, North Carolina, gave us sensitive insights concerning end-of-life issues.

David Yankelevitz, M.D., of Weill Medical College—an essential contributor to the research described in this book on early screening for lung cancer with spiral CT—made helpful comments on chapters concerning that work.

Our thanks to the following individuals who graciously agreed to let us quote from or adapt their work: Kerry S. Courneya, Ph.D., of the University of Alberta in Canada; Karl Fagerstrom, Ph.D., of Fagerstrom Consulting in Sweden; and Rabbi Harold Kushner, of Temple Israel in Natick, Massachusetts. We also thank the Canadian Lung Association for permission to use its material for people concerned about friends who smoke; PRR, Inc. of Melville, New York, for permission to use the illustrations for exercises; and the American Society for Clinical Oncology for permission to quote from their guidelines for follow-up care.

We were very fortunate to have the assistance and support of the following staff members of ALCASE, the Alliance for Lung Cancer Advocacy, Support, and Education:

Scott Rivers reviewed the entire manuscript with great sensitivity to patient needs and concerns. He also helped us contact lung cancer survivors to interview for the book.

Jan Healy provided helpful comments on the manuscript and expanded our horizons with her excellent suggestions for topics to add.

Anne Thompson, Betty Layne, D.D.S. and Nadine Jelsing provided valuable input with their comments on early drafts of the book.

Another tireless lung cancer advocate who helped us enormously is Karen Parles, founder of Lungcanceronline.org, a superb resource for anyone who needs information about this disease. Karen reviewed the entire book with great care and made many important suggestions for improving it.

This book has been enriched tremendously by the words of lung cancer survivors and their loved ones, as well as others touched by this disease. Our warm appreciation to the following people for sharing their stories with our readers in the hope of helping others, even when that meant discussing painful and difficult experiences. (In some cases we can thank them only with first names or pseudonyms to preserve their privacy.)

Marcel Baruch, Ben, Brian, Carolyn, Jim Clapp, Ken and Barbara Giddes, Glenn, Howard and Shirley Goller, Estrea Dworkin Janoson, Joanne, Anita Johnston, Joyce, Jules, Kathryn, Alan Landers, Larry, Lisa, Donna Maloney, Michael, Pat, Phil, Phyllis, Donna Purple, Selma Rosen, Tina St. John, Alice Trillin, John Troy, Tracy Walter, Carol and Doug Wilson. And special thanks, for all their extra efforts on our behalf, to Estrea Dworkin Janoson, Anita Johnston, and Donna Purple.

We've enjoyed considerable support from associates in the publishing world. Our thanks to the splendid staff at W. W. Norton for their efforts in producing this book—and for their responsiveness to our suggestions. Our able editor, Amy Cherry, reviewed the manuscript with care. We are grateful for her unfailing cheerfulness as well as her impressive expertise. Her assistant, Lucinda Bartley, provided valuable assistance of many kinds. The text benefited from the copyediting of Ted Johnson. And our appreciation to the talented people in production. Nancy Palmquist, Andy Marasia, Sue Carlson, and Adrian Kitzinger managed to turn a typewritten manuscript into an attractive book.

Wendy Weil, our agent, has buoyed us with her enthusiasm for this project. It was a pleasure to work with our talented illustrator, Robin Jensen, who produced the drawings for the book on remarkably short notice. Four excellent writers—Anita Bartholomew, Pat McNees, Sally Wendkos Olds, and Barbara Sofer—read portions of the book at various stages; their helpful comments improved it considerably. William Lockeretz gave the entire manuscript a careful review, offering many valuable suggestions. Janice Hopkins Tanne provided a steady flow of up-to-the-minute clippings from medical journals. Members of the ASJA forum and the Write It Right forums on Compuserve answered vexing questions about grammar and wording. Our gratitude to all of them (especially Dodi Schultz) for their wisdom.

Our work was facilitated in many ways by the competent and patient assistance of Robin Barnstead, Jo An Loren, and Mark White of McCarthy Medical. Heather Blades and Carolyn Hill of Weill Medical College also provided valuable logistical support.

   With heartfelt thanks to all—
   Claudia Henschke
   Peggy McCarthy
   Sarah Wernick

PART I

The Changing Face of Lung Cancer

CHAPTER 1

New Information That Could Save Your Life

by Claudia Henschke

Michael is a vigorous man in his late 50s who looks about a decade younger. He's just had a CT scan at New York Hospital, where I am chief of the Division of Chest Imaging. This painless twenty-second scan could save his life—and it could save as many as 100,000 lives every year in the United States alone.

A CT scan (also called a CAT scan) is similar to an x-ray, but it reveals a great deal more. My research, conducted with colleagues at Cornell University and New York University, has shown that a CT scan can find lung cancer before the patient has any symptoms, while the disease is still treatable and—yes—curable. Michael read about our research in the *New York Times*. Both his parents died young, and Michael is vigilant about his health. He called my office for an appointment.

The test is quick and simple. Michael lay down on the scanning table. He 'took a deep breath and held it. Silently, the table glided through the scanning doughnut—a vertical ring about as big as a tractor tire. Before he exhaled, the device had already created detailed images of his lungs.

Now Michael is in my office waiting for the results. He has no symptoms of any illness, let alone a deadly disease like lung cancer. I know from his medical folder that he watches his diet. Most mornings he jogs before work. But years ago, starting in his early teens, Michael smoked more than a pack a day. He quit in his mid-40s, shortly after his father's fatal heart attack. Unfortunately, damage may remain, even all these years later, and that concerns me.

When I bring up images of his lungs on my computer screen, I see something I don't want to see. The large oval on the right—his left lung—is

1

black, as it's supposed to be. But on the bottom of the left oval is an ominous irregularly shaped shadow of gray. Such a shadow may be caused by the inflammation and excess fluid of pneumonia. I hope that's what it is.

I question Michael about possible symptoms: "Have you had any fever or chills in the past few weeks?"

"No," he responds eagerly. "I've been feeling great." My heart sinks. That's the wrong answer. How I wish I could tell Michael that everything is fine, or even that he has pneumonia. Though pneumonia can be serious, usually we can cure it with antibiotics. Instead, I must break the news that he needs further tests and that he could have lung cancer.

Lung cancer is one of medicine's most dreaded diagnoses. The current five-year survival rate is only 14 percent. It's the leading cancer killer, by a wide margin. According to American Cancer Society statistics, the disease will claim about 157,000 lives this year in the United States. That's 28 percent of all deaths from cancer, more than the toll from colon cancer, prostate cancer, and breast cancer put together. But now there's hope that lung cancer's terrifying statistics can change.

Ordinarily, a lung cancer tumor isn't discovered until it causes symptoms. By then, the tumor usually is about the size of a small orange and the cancer probably has already spread. An x-ray can reveal a grape-size lump. But a CT scan can find tiny tumors no bigger than a grain of rice. When lung cancer is found and treated early, five-year survival rates soar from a dismal 14 percent to 70 percent or even higher. We believe that when the promise of early detection becomes a widespread reality, annual lung cancer deaths could be cut in half. When that happens, the total number of cancer deaths also will drop significantly. Indeed, early detection of lung cancer promises to have a greater impact on the war against cancer than any other single factor on the horizon.

The study that Michael read about followed 1,000 smokers and ex-smokers. We checked their lungs with chest x-rays and CT scans. In this initial screening, CT found twenty-seven tumors, twenty-three of which were still at an early stage. X-rays identified only four of these early cancers. Our findings were published in the British medical journal *Lancet* in 1999, and made headlines worldwide.

Michael will need several additional tests to determine if the shadows on his CT scan are lung cancer. If so, he can be greatly encouraged by the fact that it was discovered so early. His chances for a full recovery are excellent.

A Personal Note from Claudia Henschke

I grew up hearing about the history of lung cancer. My father, Dr. Ulrich Henschke, was a physicist and radiation oncologist whose distinguished career began in Berlin in the 1930s. One of his colleagues made the historic finding that the fatal "mountain sickness" of Czechoslovakian miners wasn't tuberculosis or some other bacterial infection, but lung cancer caused by exposure to natural radon in the mines. At the time, there were only a few hundred documented cases of lung cancer in the entire world. Today, it's astonishing to think that lung cancer was a rare disease just sixty years ago.

My father was a prolific inventor. As a child, I loved to watch him experiment in our kitchen. I remember him stirring a bubbling spaghetti pot filled with long, slender nylon tubes. Imbedded in the tubes were tiny gold pellets. When the tubes became soft from the heat, he twisted them around doorknobs to see if the pellets moved. From these endeavors came medical devices that could be implanted in patients and used to deliver radioactive seeds directly to a tumor.

When I was a teenager, I earned money by reading radiation badges for my father, checking the exposure of workers in his laboratory. During medical school and my residency in radiology, I looked forward to working with him as a doctor. Sadly, that was not to be. In those years he traveled all over the world, helping to set up cancer centers. On one such trip to Africa in 1980, he died in a plane crash. He left a rich legacy: the radiotherapy programs he established, the students he trained, and the medical devices that bear his name and are used to this day.

Deadly Myths about Lung Cancer

CT scans can transform the prognosis for men and women at risk for lung cancer. But they are not enough. People are distressingly ignorant about this disease—and what they don't know could kill them.

Myth #1: Only Smokers Are at Risk.

FACT: Most people diagnosed with lung cancer today are not current smokers, but ex-smokers. When smokers quit, their risk of lung cancer slowly drops over a fifteen-to-twenty-year period, but it remains elevated. Even if all smokers stubbed out their last cigarette tomorrow, lung cancer would remain at epidemic levels for at least the next two decades.

Moreover, each year about 26,000 Americans who *never* smoked learn they have lung cancer. Some were exposed to toxic chemicals or asbestos at work; others inhaled pollutants (including secondhand tobacco smoke and radon) at home. Genetic factors may have made them particularly vulnerable. The specific cause is not always known. We don't often hear about non-smokers with lung cancer, but annual deaths in this forgotten category exceed those from leukemia.

Myth #2: If You Smoke, the Damage Is Done, So There's No Point Quitting.

FACT: Your body has a remarkable ability to repair itself. Even if you've smoked for decades, your immune system has a chance to correct some of the damage if you stop now. Moreover, you'll prevent further harm. A University of California researcher who reviewed the statistics found that smokers who quit after age 70 lived longer than those who kept on puffing. Quitting helps even if you already have lung cancer: you will respond better to treatment and reduce the odds that cancer will reappear. And of course you'll also reduce your risk of heart disease and other smoking-related illnesses.

Myth #3: Women Need Not Worry about Lung Cancer.

FACT: Lung cancer is by far the leading cancer killer of women. According to American Cancer Society statistics, each year nearly 70,000 women will die from lung cancer in the United States—about 28,000 more than will die of breast cancer.

Tracy, a lifelong nonsmoker, was diagnosed at age 33. She recalls:

I had a funny coworker who made me laugh a lot. I noticed that my laugh felt different and sounded different—it had a crackly, rattly sound. I went to my doctor to check it out and she referred me to a lung specialist.

I was given an x-ray and a CT scan. At first they assumed I had pneumonia, and I was treated with antibiotics. But after a month, there was no improvement. Then they thought it might be a fungal infection.

Finally, Tracy had a bronchoscopy, a test in which the lungs are examined directly. She returned to the lung specialist to get the results:

This doctor is a wonderful, sympathetic person. I was sitting in his office with my two-year-old daughter crawling all over my lap while he read the report. His mouth fell wide open. He told me that I had cancer, and I could tell he was shocked.

Myth #4: The First Sign of Lung Cancer Is Coughing Up Blood.

FACT: Coughing up blood is the lung cancer symptom we've all heard about. Though this may happen as the disease progresses, it's rarely the *first* signal that something is wrong. More common early symptoms are breathlessness and fatigue. Joyce realized only later—after she was diagnosed with lung cancer at age 56—that she and her doctor had missed several significant signs:

I was exhausted. But I was working full-time as a social worker and moonlighting one or two weekend days each month. My first thought was: I don't need that second job. Also, I would be awakened with pain in my chest and down my left arm. I assumed it was my heart. My internist checked me and said, "Your heart is fine. You must have pulled a muscle."

Finally, a colleague gave her a pointed warning that sent her back to the doctor for a more thorough checkup:

We had walked up a flight of stairs. She said to me, "Joyce, you need to go to the doctor. You're slender and work out, but you're short of breath. I'm overweight and out of shape, but I'm not huffing and puffing."

Myth #5: If You're Diagnosed with Lung Cancer, the Situation Is Hopeless.

FACT: Lung cancer is one of the most undertreated cancers because many patients—and even doctors—don't realize that treatment is helpful at every stage. Even if the disease has advanced, treatment can relieve symptoms, improve the quality of life, and extend life.

All too many lung cancer patients are told, "Nothing can be done."
This is almost never true.

———

The oncologist on call came to me and said, "The diagnosis is
confirmed; it is lung cancer." He was wearing a dark blue suit. When
he said this, he held his hands in front of him and turned his head
down. I could only liken it to a funeral director trying to be sensitive
to the family. I asked him, "Isn't there anything you can do?" He
said, "There's nothing we can do."

My wife took over. Everyone should have an advocate like my
wife. It's because of her that I'm alive today. I was saying, "I'm going
to die," but she was saying, "No, we're going to beat this thing." She
got rid of the funeral director doctor and found a physician who said,
"I'll do everything I can to save you."
—*Glenn*

———

How This Book Can Help

I want to introduce my coauthor, Peggy McCarthy. Peggy is the founder of the only nonprofit organization operating internationally that is devoted solely to helping people at risk for and living with lung cancer: the Alliance for Lung Cancer Advocacy, Support, and Education (ALCASE). Through ALCASE's telephone hotline, conferences, and other programs, Peggy has met thousands of lung cancer patients. We've written most chapters of this book together, but some specialized ones separately. You'll also hear from lung cancer survivors who share their experiences and their hard-won expertise.

Here's what this book provides:

A Blame-Free Approach to Smokers

Lung cancer patients often meet with condemnation instead of compassion. Sometimes they're tormented by self-criticism. We want to clear the air about guilt, right from the start. Peggy—a former smoker herself—tackles this issue forcefully in Chapter 2.

Basic Information about the Lungs and Cancer

Your lungs bring life-giving oxygen into your body. We'll explain how they work and list simple signs—such as needing extra pillows at night—that could reveal a hidden respiratory problem. We'll also describe how cancer develops and how the body's immune system fights back. You'll gain a deeper understanding of the latest approaches to cancer treatment, such as anti-angiogenesis drugs that kill tumors by cutting off their blood supply.

Lifesaving News about Early Detection

I will give you the very latest information about CT screening and other techniques for early diagnosis. You'll find out if you need to be screened; I'll tell you where to go for testing and what to expect.

―――――

I went to my doctor because I was experiencing severe abdominal cramps. He sent me for a CT scan of the abdomen and pelvis.

After the scan, the radiologist had a strange look on his face. He said, "Nothing is wrong," but it was clear from his face that something was wrong. He wanted to take a CT scan of my chest. I'm thinking: What does that have to do with my abdomen?

I returned to my doctor to follow up. I had an acute case of constipation, which explained the cramps. But there was a small nodule on my left lung, which turned out to be malignant.

I was very lucky. Because the cancer happened to be at the very bottom of my lung, it could be seen on the CT scan of my abdomen. The doctors said my stomachache saved my life.

—Estrea

―――――

Risk Factors and How to Beat Them

Smoking is by far the leading cause of lung cancer. And it's not just ordinary cigarettes. You'll learn about the risks of cigars, marijuana, and the exotic cigarettes—bidis and kreteks—that have become alarmingly popular among teenagers. If you smoke, Peggy has encouraging news: new approaches make it a lot easier to give up cigarettes without gaining weight.

Other factors play a role in lung cancer too. We'll help you assess—and minimize—your other risks, including environmental and workplace carcinogens. We'll also suggest ways to boost your immune system. You'll learn about current research on vitamins that seem to protect against the disease.

The Best Diagnostic Strategies

My group at Cornell, along with other teams from leading cancer centers throughout North America, Europe, and Asia, are conducting additional clinical studies on early detection of lung cancer by CT scan. We expect this test soon will be as routine for lung cancer as are tests for early detection of breast, cervical, colorectal, and prostate cancers. But until that happens, most lung cancers will be discovered only when symptoms appear. You need to know about the seemingly minor changes that could signal lung cancer. We'll provide essential information about diagnostic tests, with important suggestions for avoiding unnecessary invasive procedures.

How to Find the Right Doctors

Peggy offers supportive advice for those first days and weeks when you're struggling to cope with the diagnosis and sharing the news with loved ones. There's much you can do for yourself, even before treatment begins. We have valuable tips on researching your disease, with a step-by-step guide to tapping online resources. We'll also tell you how to assemble a first-rate medical team and how to work effectively with your doctors.

The Latest on Treatment

This book presents up-to-the-minute information about lung cancer surgery, radiation therapy, and chemotherapy—with glimpses at promising new approaches still under investigation. Peggy offers many patient-tested suggestions for making treatment more tolerable.

———

I tell everyone: Don't be afraid of chemotherapy. The enemy is the cancer, not the chemo. It's not like it was twenty years ago. We've all

thrown up, been constipated, suffered diarrhea. You won't experience anything you haven't experienced from some other cause.
—*Anita*

Lung cancer therapy is advancing rapidly. We'll tell you how to join research projects that are testing the treatments of the future. The chapter on complementary and alternative options will help you sort through the possibilities to find measures that are truly helpful.

Advice on Living Well with Lung Cancer

This book addresses the emotional and practical concerns of survivors who wonder: Will my cancer return? We'll explain what tests you need to monitor your health after treatment is over.

Lung cancer and its treatments can produce difficult symptoms. But we'll tell you how to remain as healthy, active, and pain-free as possible. We'll also discuss the practicalities, including how to get what you're entitled to from your insurance company or HMO. If you have lung cancer, you know that your disease affects your loved ones too. The book includes a chapter from Peggy just for caregivers.

In the final chapter Peggy offers practical and compassionate assistance for people facing limited time. It's never too late for hope, for joy, and for meaningful accomplishments. For John, there's hope that an experimental drug will shrink the tumors that didn't respond to previous chemotherapy. Meanwhile, he's planning for the future:

> *I had a health care proxy done; I've arranged to go to a hospice when the time comes that I can't do for myself. I think anyone over forty-five should have these things in order. When you're handed a terminal diagnosis, getting things squared away frees you to add to the quality of your life. I went back to college. I'm also getting my first art show together, and I'm looking forward to that.*

The lung cancer epidemic has been a silent one. Celebrities haven't staged lavish benefit concerts; patients haven't marched on Washington to demand a cure. This is the cancer that no one talks about. We wrote this book to break the silence and explode the myths—and to offer hope to everyone at risk for and affected by this terrible disease.

Running on Hope

Jim, then 42, was diagnosed in March 1997 with inoperable lung cancer. "How long do I have?" Jim asked his doctor. The dismal reply: "Maybe as little as six months, but certainly no more than two and half years."

Another doctor offered hope. That summer—after chemotherapy to shrink the tumor—Jim's left lung was removed. Then he endured another round of chemotherapy. Jim recalls the worst days of his treatment:

> *My bathroom is on the second floor. I'd climb upstairs to urinate and when I got to the bathroom I didn't have enough energy to stand like a man—I had to sit down.*

After Jim finished chemotherapy, he made a commitment to himself to walk every day. Gradually, his strength returned. One day he tried a twenty-five-yard jog:

> *I didn't have a heart attack; I didn't fall down. I was puffing a little, but I could do it, damn it. When I got home, my wife wanted to know why I had a big grin on my face.*

In the lung cancer support group Jim attended, people used to say,

"We'll never have a race for a cure, because we can't run." Jim took that as a challenge. In the spring of 1999 he decided to train for a marathon. But first he checked with his doctor.

> My pulmonologist looked at me as if I was nuts. He said, "I don't have any experience with this. I can't get my other patients to walk. But you seem to be doing well, so go ahead."

Jim figured out how to pace himself with just one lung. He'd run as long as he could, then slow to a walk to catch his breath. All through the summer, he ran in the middle of the night to avoid the debilitating Virginia heat. He says:

> Training for a marathon is like having cancer treatment. You're pushing yourself through pain. There's a sense of being alone, and there's uncertainty. Maybe I'd go through all this and not finish.

In October 1999, Jim Clapp ran the Marine Corps Marathon, completing the twenty-six-mile course in just over seven hours. More significant than the time was the date. When he was diagnosed, he'd been given at most two and a half years—thirty months—to live. Jim was in his thirty-first month as a lung cancer survivor when he crossed the finish line.

CHAPTER 2

Clearing the Air about Guilt

by Peggy McCarthy

"I've just been diagnosed with lung cancer and I need to talk to someone." The woman's voice sounded hoarse and rough, and she was choking back tears.

As founder of ALCASE—the Alliance for Lung Cancer Advocacy, Support, and Education—I've fielded hundreds of calls from lung cancer patients and their loved ones. This was one of the saddest.

"I know you've had shocking news," I told the woman sympathetically. I introduced myself and waited for her to do the same. "I don't want to give you my name," she said. "I don't want anyone to know I have lung cancer." She was crying, struggling to speak. "I've been smoking for more than fifty years, ever since I was sixteen. I caused this myself and I'm so ashamed. I'm not going to tell anyone—not my husband, not my children, and not any of my friends."

I've never experienced the anguish that this woman felt when she heard the words "You have lung cancer." But as a former smoker, I understand her guilt. Though I quit more than thirty years ago, I know I'm still at risk. I feel even worse about exposing my two daughters to secondhand smoke when they were young.

I talked with the anonymous caller for more than an hour. She was at a pay phone, and every three minutes I'd hear more coins drop. For the past six months she'd been troubled by a chronic cough. At a routine medical checkup two weeks earlier, she had mentioned the cough to her internist, who referred her to a pulmonologist—a physician who treats diseases of the lungs. He took a chest x-ray, then delivered the news. There were tumors in both lungs, and surgery was impossible. He saw no point in further tests or treatment, claiming they would only make her sicker. His only advice was: "Go home, get your affairs in order, and enjoy whatever time you have left."

I urged her to see a lung cancer specialist to confirm the diagnosis and plan treatment; I described several patients who were doing quite well three or more years after a similar diagnosis. I tried to persuade her to let her family and friends know what she was facing, because she would need their support. And I told her what I'd told myself: "You smoke because you're addicted to cigarettes. Please don't be angry with yourself. Turn that anger toward the tobacco companies for deliberately manufacturing a deadly and addictive product."

There were warnings on cigarettes; I could have stopped smoking. But you don't read the warnings. You figure, if it was really so bad, they wouldn't let you buy it.
—Anita

One of the tragedies of lung cancer is that on top of everything else, patients often feel overwhelmed by guilt. And sometimes they're stung by criticism from family, friends, and even health care providers. Unfortunately, many people view lung cancer as a lesson in the wages of sin.

The senseless guilt and stigma attached to this disease are not merely sad; they're deadly. In part because of pervasive negative feelings about smokers (and even ex-smokers), many lung cancer patients aren't offered the aggressive treatments routinely provided for those with other types of cancer. And guilt-ridden patients don't demand measures that could prolong and improve their lives. We need to confront these attitudes—and to change them.

After my diagnosis, I asked an oncologist what I could do to prevent a recurrence. He said, "Quit smoking." I said, "I did that fifteen years ago."
—Estrea

A Personal Note from Peggy McCarthy

In the late 1980s, my medical education company, McCarthy Medical Marketing, developed a comprehensive resource guide for cancer survivors. As I reviewed the first draft, I noticed that something was missing: we offered nothing for people with lung cancer. My staff had been unable to find a single resource. I sent them back to the telephones. Finally, a doctor in Chicago produced a name: Mort Leibling. I called him.

Mort had lost one lung to cancer in 1979 at age 67. Surgery had left him breathless, fatigued, and in constant pain, but his doctor could offer no help. Unwilling to give up, Mort consulted fitness experts. With their assistance he developed a series of exercises so effective that he eventually competed in Senior Olympics walking events. Mort had published his regimen in a brochure, which he distributed for free to doctors and patients.

Our guide listed Mort and his brochure, the sole resource for people with lung cancer. Over the next few years, Mort and I talked on the telephone regularly. In 1992 I finally met this man whom I'd come to admire tremendously. His life was not going well at that point. He told me the heartbreaking story of his wife's death the previous year, his depression afterward, and the decline in his health. He said, "I know I'm not going to live much longer. Would you be willing to continue what I started?" With tears streaming down our cheeks, we began to plan.

Mort died in December 1994. One month later, I founded ALCASE—the Alliance for Lung Cancer Advocacy, Support, and Education, the first nonprofit organization dedicated solely to people with lung cancer. Our newsletter bears the name of Mort's exercise program: Spirit and Breath.

My lung cancer education has been continued by the hundreds of other patients and their family members to whom I've talked over the years. Some were friends before their diagnosis; many became friends afterward. Their experiences, which they have shared so generously, have inspired and guided my activities as a lung cancer advocate.

Accusatory Loved Ones

Another haunting ALCASE call came from a woman whose husband had just been diagnosed with lung cancer. She said: "I've been telling him for twenty-five years to quit smoking, but he ignored me. Now he's got lung cancer and I don't feel even a tiny bit sorry for him. I'm just damn mad." I felt so sad for both of them. Anger—on the part of family members as well as patients—is a common reaction to any cancer diagnosis. This unhappy woman had just retired; she had been looking forward to enjoying her life. Her resentment was understandable.

I talked to her about the losses she was facing: "Instead of doing fun things together, you'll be nursing someone who's very ill, who may be dying. It's normal to grieve, and anger is part of the grieving process." I told her that her husband would experience similar feelings. I urged her to speak with an experienced counselor to help both of them cope with these powerful emotions.

Lung cancer is thought of as something you bring on yourself. I could see that in the faces of some people when I told them. One person said to me, "You smoked like a chimney—what did you expect?" I thought that was cruel, but I let it go. I'm more interested in living than in the small stuff.
—Glenn

Unsympathetic Health Care Providers

Even experienced medical professionals find it difficult to tell a patient that he or she has lung cancer. Many doctors manage to find gentle and comforting words. But all too often, ALCASE callers tell us that physicians make unsympathetic, accusatory comments, such as "Well, that's what happens when you smoke."

The decision to smoke is nearly always made during adolescence. Kids are hooked by alluring advertisements, peer pressure, and the sense of invulnerability that's part of being young. Because cigarettes are addictive, it's much harder to give up smoking than it is to abandon other risky youthful behavior.

Most experts believe that at least half of all cancers could be prevented by wiser behavior. Moreover, cancer is not the only serious illness that we bring upon ourselves. Have a look at the table below, which shows the ten leading causes of death in the United States. *All* of them are at least partly linked to poor lifestyle choices or personal negligence. Yet these carry little or no stigma. Neither should lung cancer.

Ten Leading Causes of Death in the United States

CAUSE OF DEATH	LIFESTYLE CONTRIBUTORS	ANNUAL TOLL
Heart disease	Smoking, overweight, poor diet, inactivity, stress	725,000
Cancer (all types)	Smoking, overweight, inactivity, excessive sun exposure, avoidable exposure to toxic chemicals	542,000
Stroke	Smoking, overweight, inactivity, stress	158,000
Chronic obstructive pulmonary disease	Smoking, avoidable exposure to toxic chemicals	113,000
Accidents	Carelessness, recklessness, and fatigue; not using seatbelts; excessive alcohol consumption	98,000
Pneumonia; flu	Failure to get immunized	92,000
Diabetes	Overweight, poor diet, inactivity, inadequate control of established diabetes	65,000
Suicide	Failure to recognize and treat depression	31,000
Kidney disease	Uncontrolled diabetes, uncontrolled high blood pressure	26,000
Liver disease	Excessive alcohol consumption, drug use	25,000

SOURCE: Based on data from National Vital Statistics Reports, vol. 48, no. 11.

A Nonsmoker's Experience

Alice Stewart Trillin was 38 when she coughed up a small clot of blood, went for a chest x-ray, and learned she had lung cancer.

> *I was young. I was healthy. I had never smoked a cigarette in my life. The doctors tried to give me explanations for the tumor and seemed embarrassed that they couldn't come up with any. I sneaked a look at my hospital chart, and found in one doctor's report on me the phrase "Patient gives the story that she never smoked." This doctor simply found it necessary to blame me for having gotten lung cancer.*

SOURCE: "For a Smoking Ban in New York City," by Alice Stewart Trillin, *New York Times*, January 24, 1987. (Quoted with the permission of the late Alice Stewart Trillin.)

Shedding the Burden of Guilt

Guilt can be useful. It's one of the mind's most powerful tools for motivating self-improvement. I've met many people whose guilt about smoking motivated them to quit and to help others quit. But excessive guilt can also create stress that interferes with efforts to stop. How can you tell if guilt is excessive? Look at the impact on your life. Healthy guilt produces positive results.

When you have lung cancer, guilt about smoking usually is destructive. It saps the energy you desperately need to heal and to cope; it makes you feel unworthy of excellent medical treatment and undeserving of love and concern. If you're troubled by guilt, or if it's impairing your relationships with family or friends, I urge you to do something about it.

Begin by acknowledging to yourself that smoking is not simply a bad habit. If it were, you could easily discard it just by putting your mind to it. Nor is smoking a simple choice, like picking chocolate over vanilla. Smoking is an *addiction*—and it's a particularly powerful addiction. Many former addicts say that it was easier to give up cocaine or heroin than cigarettes. You didn't choose to become addicted. Try to separate normal regret and sadness from the more negative feelings of self-criticism and blame.

What if you are still encumbered by guilt? Sometimes it's helpful to discuss the issue with other smokers or former smokers, who may have similar feelings. Find sympathetic people to talk to—family members, friends, an ALCASE volunteer—or join a support group such as Nicotine Anonymous. If these measures don't make you feel better, I hope you will seek help. You might consult a mental health professional, such as a social worker or psychologist. Or you could talk to a religious or spiritual adviser. Look for someone who understands tobacco issues. A smoking cessation clinic might be able to make a recommendation.

———

How could I have guilt? I was a little girl born into a family and a society that encouraged me to smoke. My older brother gave me my first puff when I was three years old. Lucy and Desi, my two favorite actors, told me to do it. Doctors in TV ads told me that it would relax me and make me feel good. I have sadness and hurt, but I don't have any guilt. It took every ounce of my strength to get that monkey off my back and keep it off.
—Selma

———

I don't know what happened to the woman I told you about at the beginning of this chapter. She never gave me her name, and I never spoke with her again. But I think of her often and hope so much that she was able to make peace with herself. She didn't deserve to have lung cancer. No one does.

PART II

The Basics

CHAPTER 3

How Your Lungs Work

The human body's most urgent need is for oxygen. We can live for days without water and weeks without food. But without oxygen, we die in minutes. The vital role of our two lungs is to draw oxygen from the air we inhale, and to expel toxic carbon dioxide. When the lungs don't perform properly, every part of the body is affected.

This chapter takes you on a guided tour of your lungs and describes how they normally function. Of special interest are the mechanisms that protect the lungs from impurities in the air. When these defenses break down or are overwhelmed by toxins, lung disease—including cancer—can result.

Lung Anatomy

Your lungs occupy the top half of your torso, the central part of your body. The bottom half contains other vital organs: your stomach, intestines, liver, kidney, and pancreas. Separating the upper and lower parts of your torso is a flat muscle called the *diaphragm*. As you breathe, the diaphragm moves up and down, acting like bellows to draw air in and push air out of your lungs.

Unlike other body parts that come in pairs, your left and right lungs are not a matched set. A normal right lung has three sections, called *lobes*. The left lung, which is slightly smaller, has only two, with a "cardiac notch" to make room for the heart. You might assume that your lungs are hollow, like two balloons. But they're filled with air tubes, air sacs, lymph nodes, and blood vessels (including **arteries**, which carry blood away from the heart, and **veins**, which return it). Each lobe is like a mini-lung. If one or more lobes are removed—which sometimes happens with lung cancer treatment—the others can sustain life. Indeed, it's possible to live with just one lobe of one lung.

The space between the two lungs is called the **mediastinum**. Tucked into this area are the heart, the **trachea** (windpipe), the **esophagus** (the long tube that runs from the throat to the stomach), and many lymph nodes. To allow your lungs to move smoothly as you breathe, a slippery membrane called the **pleura** covers the inside of your chest cavity; it also covers and separates the lobes (this part is called the **visceral pleura**).

Anatomy of the Chest and Lungs

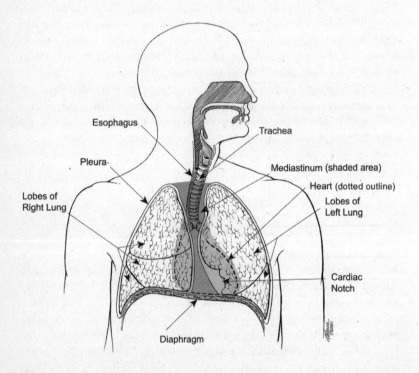

How You Breathe

Approximately one pint of air enters your body each time you inhale. A few seconds later, the same amount leaves as you exhale. In that brief time, your respiratory system moves oxygen into your bloodstream and extracts carbon dioxide. This transfer is made deep inside your lungs.

The network of airways in your lungs resembles an upside-down tree. Air travels through your nose or mouth and down your trachea. In the middle of your chest, the trachea divides into two *bronchi* (large airways), left and right, and each enters a lung at a point called the *hilum*. The two bronchi subdivide into a total of five branches, one for each lung lobe—three to the right and two to the left. Inside the lobes, the air enters progressively smaller and more delicate branches called *bronchioles*. The bronchioles end in clusters of microscopic air sacs, the *alveoli* (pronounced al-VEE-oh-lie). The walls of these sacs are very thin and fragile, but elastic. They expand like tiny balloons as the air reaches them. Healthy lungs contain more than 300 million alveoli. Though each one is too small to see with the naked eye, the combined surface area of their walls is about the size of a tennis court. This is where oxygen and carbon dioxide get transferred.

Meanwhile, your heart is pumping blood through your body via a network of blood vessels. They branch into smaller and smaller vessels, just as the air passages do. The very smallest blood vessels, called capillaries, surround the alveoli. Oxygen moves through the thin walls of the alveoli and into the capillaries. Oxygen-rich blood leaves the lungs and flows to the heart, which pumps it to the rest of the body.

As your hardworking cells receive oxygen, they discharge carbon dioxide and other toxic waste products into the bloodstream. Disposing of these wastes is just as important as providing oxygen. Carbon dioxide passes from the capillaries into the alveoli. You exhale to get rid of it. Then you inhale fresh air, and the whole process begins again.

The average person, sitting quietly, breathes about ten to fifteen times per minute. But suppose you jump up and sprint to catch a bus. As soon as you become more active, you require more oxygen; you also need to expel more carbon dioxide. Sensors in your brain detect the change and immediately direct the diaphragm to work harder. Your breathing becomes faster and deeper. If your lungs are healthy, you have plenty of reserve capacity and can easily meet these extra demands.

As You Breathe

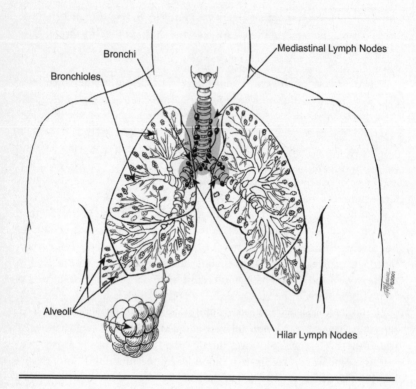

Bronchi

Mediastinal Lymph Nodes

Bronchioles

Alveoli

Hilar Lymph Nodes

Mechanisms That Protect Your Lungs

Your lungs are uniquely vulnerable. Unlike other internal organs, your delicate breathing passages are directly exposed to air and all the pollutants it contains. Several defense mechanisms are designed to protect them as much as possible.

Whenever you cough, sneeze, or clear your throat, you're guarding your lungs from environmental contaminants. Mucus—a sticky fluid secreted by cells in the lining of your nose and bronchial tubes—traps the germs, dirt, and other unwanted particles you inhale. This gunk is swept up into your throat by microscopic hair-like *cilia* that grow from the airway walls. Though you're probably not aware of it, you swallow frequently throughout the day. This sends mucus and bits of debris to your digestive tract for disposal.

Another line of defense is the lymphatic system, part of the body's *immune system*, which guards against infection and disease. *Lymph*, a fluid rich in different types of *leukocytes* (white blood cells), bathes all the tissues of the body, including the lungs. Leukocytes are an army against disease, including cancer. Some leukocytes manufacture antibodies that attack germs; others gobble up and destroy different menaces, from irritating particles to abnormal precancerous cells.

Lymph circulates through the body via a network of *lymphatic vessels* that is similar to and intertwined with the network of blood vessels. This network is dotted with *lymph nodes*, which act as filters to remove anything that could harm the body. Lymph nodes are found throughout the lungs and in the mediastinum. Cancer can spread via the lymphatic system. That's why the diagnostic process includes an examination of lymph nodes.

When Defenses Break Down

Our lungs are designed to guard against occasional invaders. But if the lungs are chronically exposed to irritants—such as tobacco smoke or other inhaled carcinogens—these natural defenses become inadequate and even counter-productive. This is what happens:

- Mucus-producing glands in the airways step up production to wash away contaminants—but they can't keep up with the continuing barrage.

- Irritants damage the cilia, which normally brush mucus and debris out of the breathing passages. Excess mucus accumulates, creating a breeding ground for infection.

- When infection occurs, the immune system sends leukocytes to join the battle, causing inflammation in the airways and alveoli. Air passages thicken and become less elastic, further impeding removal of excess mucus.

These combined effects of chronic irritation produce the symptoms typical of ordinary respiratory illness, such as breathing difficulty and coughing. Another possible consequence is *pneumonia*, an infection of the lungs. Antibiotics can treat pneumonia, but it is likely to recur if smoking or other irritation persists. Over time, two serious lung diseases may develop: chronic bronchitis in the airways, and emphysema, which affects the alveoli.

Chronic Bronchitis

This condition starts with irritation of the airways, inflammation, and increased mucus production—conditions that increase vulnerability to infection. Repeated infections lead to scarring, which narrows air passages further. Breathing becomes a struggle. The walls of the bronchi, the larger airways, are made from sturdy cartilage. But the smaller bronchioles, which don't contain cartilage, may collapse from the effort to breathe. The result of narrowed and collapsed airways is shortness of breath and fatigue, which can become severe as chronic bronchitis progresses.

Emphysema

The irritants that cause chronic bronchitis also affect the alveoli. These tiny sacs become less elastic, so they are less able to move air in and out of the lungs. In emphysema, the walls between alveoli break down, creating larger spaces with much less surface area. This means that the alveoli become less efficient at transferring oxygen and carbon dioxide to and from the bloodstream. Symptoms include a constricted feeling in the chest and shortness of breath, even at rest. Emphysema sufferers often describe themselves as "air-hungry."

Smoker's Cough

Many smokers begin the morning with a hacking cough. Here's why: Smoking increases mucus production. Hair-like cilia in the airways are supposed to sweep mucus up to the throat so it can be swallowed, but smoking impairs cilia action. Overnight, when smoking stops, the cilia recover somewhat and begin to move accumulated mucus up the airways. The smoker awakens with air passages clogged with mucus. Repeated coughing is needed to remove it.

Why Lung Disease May Make Your Ankles Swell

Lung disease can increase pressure in the blood vessels of the lungs, a condition called *pulmonary hypertension*. When you have pulmonary hypertension, blood backs up in veins elsewhere in the body. Excess fluid leaks into tissues and—thanks to gravity—pools in the ankles, causing them to swell.

Chronic Obstructive Pulmonary Disease (COPD)

When a person has both chronic bronchitis and emphysema—as often happens, especially in smokers—the condition is called *chronic obstructive pulmonary disease (COPD)*. COPD is the fourth-leading cause of death in the United States, claiming over 100,000 lives per year.

It's important to know about these conditions for two reasons. First, there is considerable overlap between the symptoms of lung cancer and those of COPD. Second, COPD is a wake-up call. The same irritants that cause chronic bronchitis or emphysema also can cause lung cancer.

Are Your Lungs Healthy?

Our lungs have so much extra capacity that if something goes wrong, we may not realize it right away. This is particularly true for people who aren't physically active. But just as it is important to be aware of an erratic heartbeat or alterations in vision, we need to be alert to subtle changes in pulmonary function—the performance of our lungs. Here are some signs to watch for:

- You're tired during the day, even though you get enough sleep.

- Climbing a flight of stairs or walking up a hill has become much harder.

- Slight exertion leaves you out of breath.

- If you're walking with a friend your own age, you have to slow down to talk.

- You're coughing more than usual.

- You've begun to make noises when you breathe.

- At night you now need extra pillows to breathe comfortably.

- Your bed partner says that your snoring has gotten worse.

- You're getting more frequent or lengthier respiratory infections.

Don't be alarmed if you notice a difference. Usually, these changes are innocuous, indicating nothing more than a cold. Or they could reflect the fact that you're out of shape and need to get more exercise. But if a problem persists, bring it to your doctor's attention just in case. In Chapter 8 we'll discuss lung cancer symptoms in more detail.

A Pulmonary Checkup

Even if you have no symptoms of lung disease, your doctor will listen to your respiratory system during a checkup, using a stethoscope pressed to your

Belly Breathing

Do you breathe too shallowly? Most adults do. Instead of filling their entire lungs, each new breath enters just the upper portion. As a result, the lungs have to work harder.

To find out if you're breathing shallowly, put one hand on your chest and the other on your belly. Then inhale and watch your midsection. Did your abdomen move forward—or did your chest and shoulders rise? If the motion was mainly in your chest and shoulders instead of in your abdomen, you're breathing shallowly.

Belly breathing (also called abdominal or diaphragmatic breathing) uses the bellows-like power of the diaphragm, the muscle under the lungs. When the diaphragm relaxes and drops down, air is drawn deep into the lungs. As the diaphragm contracts and rises, carbon dioxide is forced out. This maximizes the exchange of air with each breath.

chest or upper back. This is called **auscultation** (listening). A trained ear can detect the presence of fluid or obstructions in the airways as you breathe. Other tests may be performed to assess any symptoms. It's important to tell your doctor about any changes in pulmonary function.

Spirometry

Spirometry uses a *spirometer*, a device that measures the volume and speed of air movement, to assess your lung power. To be tested, you breathe into a spirometer while clips hold your nose shut. The two measurements most commonly made are:

- *FVC* (forced vital capacity), the total volume of air you can expel in one full exhalation

- *FEV₁* (forced expiratory volume in one second), the amount of air you can expel in one second

The results are compared to standard scores for someone of your age, sex, and height. Abnormally low scores could mean that your airways are obstructed.

Practice belly breathing to get yourself into better breathing habits:

- Lie down. Place your hands on your abdomen with your thumbs on either side of your navel.

- As you inhale, push your belly out.

- When you exhale, squeeze your abdominal muscles in, and push them back toward your spine. Your chest and shoulders should not move at all.

Once these muscle movements are familiar, try them in a standing position. Belly breathing is also an excellent stress reducer. Many people feel stronger and healthier when they make the switch from chest to belly breathing and use their lungs more effectively.

Spirometry: A Simple, Inexpensive— and Underused—Test

Blood pressure is taken routinely during medical examinations to check the heart. Many pulmonary experts believe that spirometry should be used similarly to evaluate lung health. The test, which can be performed in just a few minutes in a doctor's office, can detect damage at a very early stage, while there is still time for corrective measures. In 2000, a consensus statement from the National Lung Health Education Program called for primary care physicians to use spirometry on all patients with respiratory symptoms, as well as on those age 45 or older who smoke.

Arterial Blood Gas Analysis (ABG)

Using a blood sample drawn from an artery, doctors can measure various indicators of lung function, including concentrations of oxygen and carbon dioxide in the blood. This indicates how well the lungs are moving oxygen into the bloodstream and extracting carbon dioxide from it.

A noninvasive (but also more limited) blood gas test is *pulse oximetry*. A sensor is attached to the finger, toe, or earlobe—places where the bloodstream is close to the surface of the skin. The sensor sends a light signal through the skin and measures how much is absorbed; this indicates how much oxygen the blood contains.

The healthier your lungs are, the less likely you are to get lung cancer. That's in part because healthy lungs have stronger defenses, and in part because smoking and other factors that cause poor lung health also increase the risk of cancer.

CHAPTER 4

When Cancer Intrudes

C ancer takes more than a hundred different forms, affecting different parts of the body and producing different symptoms. But the disease always begins the same way: with genetic damage that permits abnormal cells to spread. This chapter explains how cancer starts. But first, you'll need to understand how genes normally guide and control our growth.

Genetic Fundamentals

Human growth is like a manufacturing process, complete with a blueprint and quality control mechanisms. The blueprint is the *genome*, the set of *genes* that provide detailed instructions for development. Each gene governs a particular trait. Genes, which are made up of *DNA (deoxyribonucleic acid)*, are organized on threads called *chromosomes*.

The entire genetic plan—approximately 30,000 genes clustered on twenty-three pairs of chromosomes—is contained in the fertilized ovum with which our life begins. This cell divides and forms two cells, each with a copy of the genome. Cell division continues, and we begin to grow. Whenever a cell divides, all the genes must be copied all over again.

Following the blueprint, new cells *differentiate:* they acquire specialized capabilities and characteristic appearances. Some differentiate into bone cells; others are destined to be part of our heart, brains, lungs, and other organs. Cell division continues and the body grows—up to a point.

The Role of the Immune System

The immune system identifies and destroys cells with genetic defects, just as it guards against germs. Individuals with compromised immune systems—such as people with AIDS or those taking drugs to prevent rejection of organ transplants—lack this potent weapon. As a result, they suffer from high rates of cancer. One focus of cancer research is looking for ways to optimize immune system functioning.

Crucial to the genetic blueprint are the instructions that limit growth. Certain genes, called *proto-oncogenes*, tell our cells to divide. But others, *tumor-suppressor genes*, halt cell division. Normally, we grow rapidly as children and adolescents. If this continued, we'd become larger and taller every year. Instead, thanks to genetic instructions, our growth slows and stops as we reach adulthood. Cells continue to divide, but just enough to replace existing cells as they become damaged or wear out and die.

Quality control is built into the genes too. Our cells are capable of spotting and correcting mistakes, including defective genes or imperfect copies of the genome. Every cell contains instructions for its own self-destruction in case it becomes infected or damaged. This suicidal process is called *apoptosis*, or *programmed cell death*. Apoptosis is also activated when cells age. At the end of each chromosome thread is a section called a *telomere*. Each time a cell divides, a piece of the telomere disappears. When it's all gone—after about forty divisions—the cell dies. If these safeguards don't function properly, cells can become immortal. Instead of dying, they continue to divide. This is the unchecked growth that characterizes cancer.

How Cancer Develops

Cancer begins with defective genes—not just a single gene, but several. These defects may be inherited; sometimes they occur for no obvious reason. But usually they result from exposure to *carcinogens*: cancer-causing chemicals, radiation, or viruses. In Chapter 6 we'll discuss the carcinogens that can cause lung cancer.

In general, the risk of cancer is greatest for people with the most exposure to carcinogens. However, not every exposed individual actually develops cancer. Some people are especially vulnerable because their natural defenses are poor.

Cells Out of Control

We don't yet know all the genetic scenarios that can lead to *carcinogenesis* (the development of cancer), but one of them—described by researchers at the Whitehead Institute for Biomedical Research in Cambridge, Massachusetts—involves defects in three types of genes. The scientists compare the changes that unleash cancer to the malfunctions that could produce a runaway car: the accelerator gets stuck; the brakes give out; and the gas tank doesn't run dry.

- **Defect #1—the stuck accelerator:** Proto-oncogenes, which stimulate cell division, turn into *oncogenes:* they're turned on and don't respond to signals to turn off. So far, about sixty different oncogenes have been identified. Among those linked to lung cancer are *ras, myc,* and *HER/2neu.*

Malignant or Benign?

Not all abnormal growth is *malignant* (cancerous). Tumors that aren't cancerous are called *benign.* The cells of a benign tumor are more differentiated than typical cancerous cells. In other words, they look and act more like normal cells. Often, benign tumors are encapsulated by connective tissue—that's why they typically have smooth edges. If these tumors grow, they usually grow relatively slowly. Unlike cancerous tumors, they do not invade surrounding tissues or spread to other parts of the body.

Nevertheless, benign tumors may need to be removed. Though they're not malignant, they can cause troubling symptoms because of their size or location. Also, there's a risk that some of their cells may become cancerous.

- **Defect #2—the defective brakes:** Tumor-suppressor genes, which are supposed to control cell division, don't function properly. One of these, called *p53*, normally senses genetic abnormalities and triggers apoptosis (programmed cell death). Abnormal p53 genes are found in most lung cancer cells.

- **Defect #3—the perpetually full gas tank:** The telomeres, which usually shorten with each cell division, instead are rebuilt by a gene that's normally deactivated. This defective gene triggers release of telomerase, an enzyme that replenishes the telomeres. Instead of dying after about forty divisions, cells become immortal.

As you can see, it's not just one genetic defect but a combination that permits cancer to develop. As we learn more about the human genome, we may be able to identify people at high risk for cancer by checking their genes.

The Grim Progression

The first sign of trouble is *hyperplasia*, or excess growth. As the damaged cells continue to divide, *dysplasia* appears—abnormal, premalignant cells that no longer look or function like their normal counterparts. Dysplastic cells can be wiped out by the immune system. But if they survive and divide, they may eventually become cancerous. In other words, the cells will not only be abnormal, they'll multiply out of control. Since these new cells are not properly differentiated, they can't perform the specialized tasks of normal cells.

The speed of a cancer's growth is measured by its *doubling time*—the time it takes for the cancer cells to divide, thereby doubling in number. Aggressive cancers, which progress rapidly, might have a doubling time of only 30 days; more indolent cells might have a doubling time of 300 or more days. Lung cancers vary; typical doubling times range from about 30 to 180 days.

As cancerous cells proliferate, they form a *tumor*, a mass of abnormal tissue. Like any other cells, these defective cells depend on the bloodstream to provide their nourishment. The tumor develops blood vessels, a process called *angiogenesis*. Now the cancer is ready to spread.

Expanding tumors may invade adjacent tissues. Also, cells from the original tumor may migrate, or *metastasize*, to other parts of the body via the bloodstream or the lymphatic system. The tumor's new blood vessels facilitate transportation. Angiogenesis happens relatively early in tumor development. That's why people with small lung tumors may already have these distant cancers (called *metastases* or *secondary tumors*). One promising experimental approach to cancer treatment involves anti-angiogenesis drugs, which interrupt blood vessel development.

When Cancer Attacks the Lungs

Lung cancer usually begins in the lining of one of the bronchial tubes or in the alveoli (air sacs). Though these tissues are designed for defense, as we described in Chapter 3, they are also vulnerable because they're directly exposed to the air, with all its impurities. Protective mechanisms can break down if bombarded by carcinogens.

Hyperplasia and dysplasia, the premalignant changes that set the stage for lung cancer, can develop over decades. If we can learn how to spot these very early changes in cells, we'll have a long opportunity to intervene and halt the process. But once cells become cancerous—and develop their own blood supply—growth is more rapid and the cells can migrate to other sites.

Cancer growth patterns vary somewhat, depending on the location in the lung. The pictures on the next two pages show the typical progression of cancer in the airways.

Types of Lung Cancer

Until now we've referred to lung cancer as if it were just one disease. But lung cancer takes different forms, each with its own appearance, typical causes, and patterns of growth. A key part of diagnosis is identifying the type of lung cancer so that appropriate treatment can be planned. Some people actually have more than one kind at once.

In the future, when we know more about the genetic basis of lung cancer, we'll probably devise a new classification system. But at the moment, lung cancers are divided into two main categories, based on the appearance of the cells: small cell lung cancer (SCLC) and non-small cell lung cancer (NSCLC).

From Healthy Tissue to Metastatic Lung Cancer

Healthy tissue
The cells that line the airways look like tall columns. Some secrete mucus, which traps harmful particles from the air. Others grow hair-like cilia, which sweep away debris.

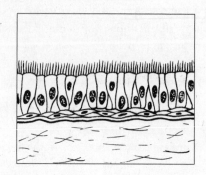

Hyperplasia
Genetic damage has occurred. Cells begin to divide more rapidly than usual. At first, the new cells appear normal or close to normal.

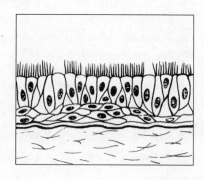

Dysplasia
Cells have de-differentiated. New cells look less like healthy airway cells; some are flat and wide instead of tall and narrow. They may lack cilia, so they can't perform their normal protective functions.

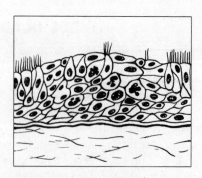

Tumor

Cells have become cancerous and have formed a tumor. Angiogenesis has begun: the tumor is developing a network of new blood vessels to sustain its growth. Depending on its location and size, the tumor may cause symptoms.

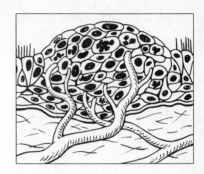

Invasive tumor

The cancer has spread beyond its original site. It may grow into the chest wall, the mediastinum (space between the lungs), or adjacent lobes of the lung.

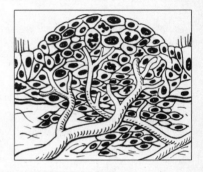

Metastatic cancer

Cancerous cells have broken off and migrated elsewhere in the body via the bloodstream or lymphatic system. Lung cancer can travel to any organ, but it most often spreads to the bones, the brain, the liver, and the adrenal glands.

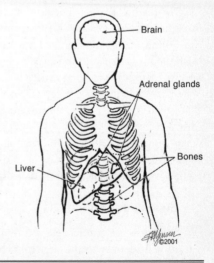

Brain

Adrenal glands

Bones

Liver

©2001

Small Cell Lung Cancer (SCLC)

SCLC is sometimes called *oat cell carcinoma*, because the cells resemble oats under the microscope. Probably about 10 to 15 percent of lung cancers are in this category.

Small cell lung cancer almost always occurs in people who have smoked. It usually develops in the bronchial airways, not on the surface of the lining but in an inner layer of tissues. This is a particularly aggressive form of cancer. Cells divide rapidly, so the disease spreads quickly. Doubling time is only about 30 days.

Non-Small Cell Lung Cancer (NSCLC)

Non-small cell lung cancer takes several different forms, which are described below. Usually NSCLC involves a single tumor. Some of these cancers grow as quickly as SCLC, but the usual doubling time is 30 to 180 days.

Adenocarcinoma

The most common kind of NSCLC is adenocarcinoma, which begins in the smaller airways or the alveoli (air sacs). The cancerous cells are tall and cylindrical; sometimes they produce mucus. Though smoking is the leading cause, this is the type of lung cancer that strikes nonsmokers most frequently.

For reasons that are not fully understood, adenocarcinoma is on the rise. One possible explanation is the switch to filtered cigarettes. Smokers tend to inhale filtered cigarettes more deeply, which allows carcinogens to reach the smaller airways and alveoli where adenocarcinoma strikes. Another relevant change is that lung cancer is increasing among women, who seem more likely than men to develop adenocarcinoma.

One distinctive type of adenocarcinoma is *bronchoalveolar carcinoma (BAC)*, which represents about 5 percent of all lung cancers. BAC causes mucus-producing cells to proliferate on the walls of the alveoli. Unlike other adenocarcinomas, BAC often involves multiple tumors rather than a single nodule. Growth is usually slow, with a dividing time of 180 days or more.

Squamous Carcinoma

Squamous carcinoma cells are thin and flat, and resemble fish scales. They usually develop in the large bronchial tubes in the center of the lungs. Squamous carcinoma occurs most frequently in men and in the elderly, and

Malignant Mesothelioma

Malignant mesothelioma is a cancer that affects the mesothelial cells. This rare disease is sometimes called lung cancer but actually is not. Mesothelial cells are found in the lining of the stomach and in the pleura, the slippery membrane that surrounds the lungs and lines the inside of the chest. Malignant mesothelioma is often caused by asbestos.

For more information:

- Contact the National Cancer Institute for its free booklet on malignant mesothelioma, which is part of the PDQ series (800-4-CANCER; *http://cancer.gov/cancerinfo/types/malignantmesothelioma*).

- See *Mesothelioma Essentials*, a web site developed by ALCASE (*http://www.mesolung.com*).

usually advances more slowly than other lung cancers. The cause nearly always is smoking. The incidence of this type of NSCLC appears to be decreasing, possibly because of the changes in smoking patterns described above.

Large Cell and Giant Cell Carcinoma

As the names imply, the cells of these cancers are relatively large. Tumors usually start in the smaller airways and grow rapidly. Large cell and giant cell carcinoma are strongly associated with smoking.

The next section of the book will discuss risk factors for lung cancer. We'll suggest many ways that you can reduce the danger.

P A R T   I I I

Beating Your Risk Factors

CHAPTER 5

Now You Can Find It Early

by Claudia Henschke

Nearly ten years ago I was visiting a friend in Florida and was involved in a really bad automobile accident. The car was totaled. Firemen pried me out of the wreckage and took me to the hospital. I had x-rays and other tests to diagnose my injuries.

The next morning, a doctor came to my room to talk to me. He said, "You have a broken pelvis and your ribs are bruised. But that's not your big problem. The big problem is that there are lesions in your lungs." He didn't use the C-word, but I said, "You're telling me I have cancer?" He said, "Yes. In both lungs." It came like a bolt out of the blue. I was totally asymptomatic. I didn't cough; I had no pain. There was absolutely no way for me to think that I had lung cancer.

—Anita

A century ago, people rarely survived for very long after any cancer diagnosis. Today, the prognosis is very different for most forms of cancer. According to National Cancer Institute statistics, the five-year survival rate for women diagnosed with breast cancer is 87 percent; for men diagnosed with prostate cancer, it's 98 percent. Colon cancer has a five-year survival rate of 62 percent. In striking contrast, the five-year survival rate for lung cancer is just under 15 percent. Lung cancer isn't more virulent than other cancers. The problem is that it's usually found too late.

Cancerous lung tumors can grow silently for years. Our lungs contain no pain fibers to alert us. Diminished functioning isn't obvious at first, because most of us have much greater lung capacity than we need in everyday life. Eventually the tumor becomes large enough to demand attention: it hinders breathing or it causes coughing or pain. But by then, the cancer probably is too advanced to cure. Most lung cancers are not discovered until they've reached this stage.

Prospects are much brighter for the lucky few whose disease is detected before it produces symptoms and before it has spread: their five-year survival rate is about 70 percent. But early lung cancers usually are found only by chance, when a person has a standard chest x-ray, CT scan, or MRI for an unrelated medical condition, as Anita did after her auto accident.

For over a decade, my colleagues and I at Weill Medical College of Cornell University in New York City have been screening people at risk for lung cancer, using low-dose CT (computed tomography) scans; CT is also called CAT (computed axial tomography). We've succeeded in detecting the disease at a much smaller size—and therefore at an earlier point in its development—than is possible with standard chest x-rays.

I expect that CT scans and other tests to detect early lung cancer will become a routine part of health care, just like mammograms and other cancer tests. But right now, lung cancer screening is controversial. Insurance plans usually don't cover it. Still, a growing number of men and women who know they're at high risk are arranging to be tested on their own. Later in this chapter I'll explain the case for lung cancer screening and offer practical advice in case you want to be checked. But first I want to tell you how the tests evolved and to explain the debate over their value.

Seeing Lung Cancer a New Way

Every Tuesday afternoon, the *thoracic* specialists at Weill College—all the surgeons, radiologists, and other doctors who treat problems of the *thorax* (chest)—gather in a conference room. On one wall hang two rows of light boxes displaying images from x-rays, CT scans, and other tests performed on patients at the hospital. We crowd around the films and discuss each case.

We have used CT scans at Weill since they were first developed in the 1970s. CT is a special way of taking an x-ray. A CT scanner takes a series of pictures; they are called "slices" because they're like the slices of a loaf of bread. The CT scanner feeds these pictures into a computer, which can reassemble the slices into a three-dimensional image of the lungs.

Early CT scanners required half an hour to scan the entire chest. One image would be taken, then the scanning table would be moved a few centimeters for the next image. Because the patient needed to breathe, the stacked images didn't always line up perfectly. Abnormal changes weren't always visible to the radiologist reading the test. But the equipment improved rapidly. In the early 1990s our institution acquired a spiral (or helical) CT. This scanner moved in a quick, smooth spiral around the patient. It took pictures of the entire chest in just twenty seconds while the patient held his or her breath. Finally we could obtain excellent CT images that included the whole lung.

After we began using the spiral CT, we occasionally found tiny **lesions** (abnormal areas) in the lungs when we hadn't suspected lung cancer but a patient's chest had been scanned for some other reason. These films provoked considerable discussion at our Tuesday conferences. None of us had ever seen lesions of this size.

At first we weren't sure what to do about them. We assumed that many were benign. But because lung cancer can be so deadly, we felt it was prudent to evaluate them further. Fortunately, there had also been advances in the techniques used to perform lung biopsies. Diagnostic surgery wasn't necessary. We could slip a very thin hollow needle between the ribs and obtain a small tissue sample to examine under the microscope. Sometimes cells in these samples appeared to be cancerous.

I'll never forget the first time one of our surgeons operated on a patient with a very small lung cancer tumor that had been discovered by spiral CT and checked with a fine needle biopsy. The doctor removed the lobe of the lung that contained the tumor and brought it to the pathology laboratory. I was waiting in the laboratory with the **pathologist,** a doctor who specializes in the analysis of tissue and fluid samples. It's standard procedure for a pathologist to determine if a tumor is cancerous. Normally, though, a surgical assistant would deliver the extracted tissue and I wouldn't be involved. But this case was different: we were all very curious about the tiny tumor.

The three of us stared at the lobe, which looked like a large sponge. Where was the cancer? The bulge of a lung cancer tumor found by chest x-ray typically is about the size of a small orange, so it's impossible to miss. The pathologist probed the lobe searching for the tumor, with no success. The surgeon picked it up and systematically examined the soft tissue with his fingers. Nothing. This was a prominent thoracic surgeon with twenty years of experience. Had he operated on the wrong lobe?

I said, "Let's see where it is on the CT." We lined up the image and the lobe. Using the CT picture as a guide, the pathologist cut into the lung. There was the tumor—a yellow lump smaller than a pea. The pathologist sliced off a thin sample, examined it under the microscope, and confirmed that it was a full-fledged cancer.

As we found and removed more of these tiny malignancies, several of us became excited about the possibility of using spiral CT scans to screen for very early lung cancer. This might sound like simple common sense—we all know that early detection is the best hope with cancer. But it isn't simple at all.

Screening is different from diagnosis. Diagnosis starts with a problem. It might be a symptom that needs to be explained, or an injury that requires assessment. But screening is performed on apparently healthy people, so we must be absolutely certain that the benefits exceed all possible risks. A spiral CT scan involves radiation exposure, but we can use a low dose for a screening test. However, in addition to detecting cancer, the scan can find harmless look-alike conditions. At the very least, these false alarms create emotional stress plus the cost and inconvenience of additional scans. Worse, a person might undergo expensive, risky, or uncomfortable diagnostic procedures— or even major surgery—for no good reason. We knew all about these problems because they had stymied an earlier generation of clinical researchers.

The Controversy over Lung Cancer Screening

You are probably familiar with early-detection tests for breast, cervical, colon, prostate, and skin cancer. So you may be puzzled to learn that lung cancer screening is not recommended by any major health organization, including the American Cancer Society, the National Cancer Institute, the American Medical Association, and many others. The explanation can be found in large studies with complex findings that were performed in the 1970s. These studies are still hotly debated. I am among those who believe that their findings were misinterpreted and that their results certainly do not apply to the medical technologies of today.

The Shadow of Previous Research

Chest x-rays have been used for about a hundred years to diagnose illness and injury. During the 1950s and 1960s, when the incidence of lung cancer began to rise and its connection with smoking became known, many doctors advised their patients who smoked to have an annual chest x-ray. As lung cancer deaths continued to soar, interest grew in a promising new technique for finding the disease early enough to save lives: *sputum cytology.* Cytology refers to the study of cells. Sputum is coughed-up material, a mixture of saliva and phlegm, the mucus secreted by the membranes that line the respiratory tract. Examination of this fluid under a microscope can reveal cancerous cells shed from the lungs and airways.

In the 1970s, large-scale investigations of sputum cytology were undertaken by three of the most outstanding medical and research institutions in the United States: Memorial Sloan-Kettering, Johns Hopkins, and the Mayo Clinic. A total of 31,360 men, all heavy cigarette smokers, participated in the three studies. (Women weren't included, because at the time their lung cancer rates were still very low.) Half of the men received regular sputum examinations; the other half—the control group—did not. The results were disappointing. Though sputum cytology detected some early lung cancers, it missed many others. Moreover, early detection didn't seem to save lives. Follow-up comparisons showed no advantage for the group that was screened.

What about chest x-rays? No comparisons were possible in the Memorial Sloan-Kettering and Johns Hopkins studies, because all participants received chest x-rays. But in the Mayo Clinic study, while the experimental group received chest x-rays and sputum exams every four months, the control group was simply advised to have "standard care." Once again, follow-up showed no benefit from screening.

These findings were baffling. Since x-rays and sputum cytology could find lung cancer at an early stage, why didn't those who were screened live longer? One explanation offered was that early diagnosis didn't affect the time of death but simply delivered the bad news sooner. Another theory was that screening led to overdiagnosis: in other words, maybe a relatively harmless type of lung cancer was detected, one that wouldn't have become life-threatening anyway.

Emerging Questions

A few skeptics took a closer look at the data and convincingly argued that the studies had serious problems that investigators had not anticipated when they designed the research. For example, a quarter of the experimental group didn't get checked as often as planned. Moreover, about half the participants in the Mayo Clinic control group had annual chest x-rays, the then-standard care at Mayo. As a result, the experimental and control groups were too similar to reveal any benefit from screening.

The overdiagnosis theory was convincingly refuted by a study of the handful of patients from the three investigations whose cancer had been found early but who did not receive surgical treatment. A total of 336 early lung cancers had been diagnosed. Most of these patients (291 out of the 336) were treated with surgery; about 70 percent of this group survived for five or more years. But 45 people did not have surgery to remove the tumor, usually because they refused treatment. Five years later, all but two of them had died of lung cancer. Clearly, the lung cancers found by x-rays and sputum cytology weren't "harmless."

Taking Another Look

Even if the recommendation against screening had been based on flawless data, it needed reexamination in the 1990s when much better detection methods—including CT scans—became available. My colleagues and I consulted Dr. Betty Flehinger, a distinguished medical statistician from the T. J. Watson Research Center in New York, who had been involved in the earlier trials. Dr. Flehinger had developed a sophisticated mathematical model for lung cancer growth. Her model predicted that annual screening with standard chest x-rays might reduce lung cancer mortality by as much as 13 percent. We asked: "What if you could detect the tumors earlier, when they were even smaller—the size a CT scan could find?" Her answer was dramatic: "The cure rate could be as high as 80 or 90 percent."

In 1992 we designed the study I mentioned in Chapter 1—called the Early Lung Cancer Action Project (ELCAP)—to evaluate the potential of CT screening for lung cancer. Over the next six years, we recruited 1,000 high-risk men and women, all of whom were age 60 or older. We checked their lungs with both a standard chest x-ray and a low-dose CT scan. The CT scans discovered lung cancer in twenty-seven of our volunteers; twenty-three of the cancers were still at the earliest stage. Only four of these very early cancers were visible on x-rays. And not one of the people we diagnosed had any symptoms of lung cancer.

Our study, published in *Lancet* in July 1999, generated considerable excitement. There had been similar investigations in Japan; we were already helping other scientists begin studies in the United States and elsewhere. We

CT and X-ray Images of the Same Lungs

These CT and x-ray images, taken at approximately the same time, show the chest of an ELCAP research volunteer who was at risk for lung cancer because of his smoking history.

CT image

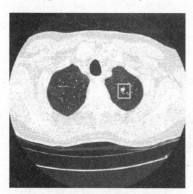

X-ray image

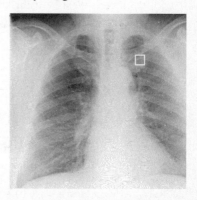

This CT image shows a "slice" of the chest. The two black ovals are the lungs: the right lung is on the left; the left lung is on the right. Normal features include the windpipe (the small black circle between the lungs) and cross sections of blood vessels and bronchi (the numerous white spots and streaks inside the lungs). The CT image also shows an abnormal area in the left lung, highlighted with a box. Subsequent tests determined that the nodule was an early lung cancer.

This x-ray image shows the lungs as dark ovals: the right lung is on the left; the left lung is on the right. Normal features include the wing-shaped collarbones and the curved horizontal stripes of the ribs. The triangular white area in the center is the heart; the smoke-like white streaks are blood vessels and bronchi. A box shows the same area of the left lung where the nodule can be seen on the CT image. However, no abnormality is visible on the x-ray.

---

decided to convene the first International Conference on Screening for Lung Cancer. In October 1999, experts from all over the world came to Weill Medical College for three days to share information. This meeting was so successful that we've held regular meetings ever since. One result is International

ELCAP, a collaborative research effort involving more than twenty institutions in the United States and throughout the world.

Meanwhile, my group at Weill (the ELCAP project) continues to gather data and refine our screening methods. In cooperation with eleven other institutions in New York State, we've started an additional study, called New York ELCAP, to validate the original ELCAP results. This time we will recruit 10,000 volunteers. We'll be using the latest CT equipment as well as an updated *screening protocol*, a systematic plan for follow-up evaluation and future testing that will be further improved throughout the study as findings develop.

Should You Have CT Screening for Lung Cancer?

You can consult a standard chart, plug in your age plus a few facts about your medical history, and learn if you should be checked for breast or colon cancer. We can't yet do that for lung cancer, though answers are evolving.

If you know you're at high risk for lung cancer (see Chapter 6 to find out), discuss CT screening with your doctor. At Weill, we accept only high-

What about Radiation Exposure from CT Scans?

Radiation can cause cancer, so it's important to limit our exposure. That's why a *low-dose* CT scan is used for screening, and that's why we recommend screening only for those at high risk for lung cancer.

When CT scans are used for diagnosis—in other words, when the purpose is to investigate symptoms or other problems rather than to check people who seem healthy—a higher-resolution image is required. Though this may entail more radiation, it's still well within the range considered safe, and the potential benefits of accurate diagnosis outweigh the very small risk.

risk people for screening. For current or former smokers, this means people age 40 and older who have a 10-pack-year history of smoking—the equivalent of a pack a day for ten years. The age requirement is based on two assumptions: first, that it typically takes about twenty years for lung cancer to evolve to a point where it's visible on CT, and second, that most people— even if they start early—don't smoke heavily as children or teenagers. We also accept people who are at risk because of exposure to secondhand smoke, air pollution, or radon, or because of occupational exposure to carcinogens.

Remember, screening is intended for apparently healthy individuals. If you have symptoms of lung cancer, diagnostic tests will be needed. See Chapter 8 for information about symptoms and diagnostic tests.

Where to Go for Testing

If you decide to be tested, be sure your test is state-of-the-art: a low-dose CT scan whose results will be interpreted by doctors experienced with CT screening for lung cancer. This will minimize the likelihood of *false positives* (test results incorrectly indicating cancer) and *false negatives* (failure to find tumors if they are present). Appropriate follow-up care is essential, as I'll explain shortly.

Here are my recommendations (see also box on page 235):

- The best testing facilities are those that are actively participating in CT screening research. You can find the current list of screening sites affiliated with ELCAP on our web sites: *http://www.nyelcap.org* and *http://www.ielcap.org*. Or call the following number for information: 212-746-1325.

- If you can't go to an affiliated screening site, have your test at a leading cancer center if possible. Check the web site of the National Cancer Institute for a list of top cancer centers (*http://www.cancer.gov/cancercenters/centerslist.html*) or call its toll-free number: 800-4-CANCER.

- If you can't be tested at one of these centers, call a university-affiliated hospital in your area.

Some independent clinics and community hospitals have begun to advertise lung cancer screening. Their ads often boast of splendid new equipment. But that's not nearly enough. Even more important is appropriate follow-up care, whether your scan finds ominous spots or seems clear. My colleagues and I have heard of patients who are subjected to needless invasive tests—and even unnecessary surgery. More commonly, they suffer pointless worry and expense, which is what happened to Phyllis:

> *I had a CT scan because I used to be a very heavy smoker and was concerned about lung cancer. I paid three hundred dollars for the test because my insurance didn't cover it.*
>
> *A week later I got a letter: "We have detected a paratracheal adenopathy." I had no idea what that meant. I was absolutely panicked. I brought the test results to my doctor. I asked her, "Should I go home and clean? I don't want to die with a dirty house."*
>
> *My doctor was very reassuring. She said, "I don't think it's cancer. However, I want you to have an MRI to find out what it is." I had the MRI; I also had another CT scan where they injected me with dye. I called a doctor friend, who gave me the names of two thoracic oncologists. I wanted a second opinion and a third opinion. I showed them all the test results and they both reached the same conclusion: it was a water-filled cyst.*
>
> *I was relieved. But I'd gone to a lot of trouble. I had to see four doctors, one of whom kept me waiting for five hours. I had three tests, including an invasive procedure with the dye. And it was expensive. My insurance picked up some of it, but the first CT scan was on me and I consulted one of the oncologists on my own.*

I haven't met Phyllis or examined her CT scan, but I was dismayed to hear about her experience. Centers like ours use a follow-up protocol—which is constantly refined on the basis of clinical research—that is designed not only to detect cancers but also to minimize unnecessary tests. Also, we know how often CT scans uncover innocuous conditions, and we've seen how frightened people become when they learn that their test has revealed something questionable. The last thing we want to do is to cause unnecessary fear. When we find an abnormality, we don't deliver the news in a letter; we always call, so we can offer immediate explanations and answer any questions. We find that most people feel greatly reassured after they speak with us.

As an ex-smoker, Phyllis had already taken the most important step toward protecting herself against lung cancer. But for current smokers, undergoing the test—and facing the possibility of lung cancer—provides excellent motivation to quit. So the best follow-up care provides smoking cessation counseling when relevant. It also includes guidance for those who have a negative scan, so they know when to schedule their next test. If you want to be tested but can't manage to visit one of the facilities recommended above, I urge you to find a radiology clinic that offers complete follow-up services.

Insurance Issues

Spiral CT is widely available; it's one of the diagnostic tests that may be given to someone whose symptoms or other test results (such as a chest x-ray) suggest possible lung cancer. However, the use of CT scans for lung cancer screening—testing people without any symptoms—is still considered experimental. This means that Medicare, most insurance companies, and most HMOs don't cover it. Expect to pay anywhere from $175 to $1,000 ($300 is typical) for a low-dose spiral CT. Fortunately, insurance nearly always covers any further tests used to evaluate a suspicious finding from a CT screening test. Also, insurance usually pays for CT scans to investigate lung cancer symptoms.

What the Test Is Like

A CT scan is painless and quick. You'll remove clothing and jewelry from the waist up, and change into a hospital gown. In the procedure room, a technician will help you lie down on the scanning "couch," which looks like a narrow examining table. The technician will tell you to take a few quick breaths to prepare. Then you'll hold your breath as the table slides through the scanning doughnut. In a matter of seconds, the scanner will take a series of pictures of

---

Do You Have Symptoms of Lung Cancer?

Fatigue? Breathlessness? Persistent coughing? Read the full list in Chapter 8, and be sure to bring any relevant symptoms to your doctor's attention before you have a screening test. You may need a *diagnostic* test, which could be slightly different. Diagnostic CT scans produce higher-resolution images than screening scans; sometimes the patient is first injected with a special dye to enhance the image. In addition, diagnostic tests usually are covered by insurance.

your chest. Computerized data from the scan is instantly transformed into detailed images that are displayed on a screen for the radiologist to check.

In the early 1990s, when we first began our research on lung cancer screening, CT scanners could take thirty pictures in a single breath-hold. A decade later, the newest scanners take 300 to 600 pictures—and they're still improving rapidly. I'm always excited to hear about the latest advances from equipment manufacturers. The more images we obtain from a test, the more detail we can see and the lower the radiation dose that is necessary for screening.

Understanding the Results

Healthy lungs look black in a CT image. When I check a scan, I'm looking for anything white that isn't a blood vessel. A cancer will be white on the image—but white areas are not necessarily cancer. Here are some of the harmless conditions I might spot:

- Scarring from a previously healed infection; scars may contain calcium deposits (called calcifications), which is why they look white on the scan

- Pneumonia, which produces fluid and inflammatory cells

- Benign tumors

- Minor congenital abnormalities

A person's first CT scan serves as a baseline. Once we've identified the permanent features of the lungs—scars, benign tumors, and other minor abnormalities—we know not to be concerned when we spot them again in future tests. If we find something new the next time, it's not necessarily cancer. With other benign conditions ruled out, the most likely explanation is pneumonia. Often people are surprised to hear that they may have pneumonia; they'll say, "But I feel perfectly fine!" Severe pneumonia can be life-threatening. However, it's quite possible to have a mild form, such as the type called "walking pneumonia," without being aware of it. CT scans are so sensitive that we can spot very small pneumonias, and even areas where mucus is accumulating but isn't infected. We prescribe antibiotics and ask the person to return in a month for a follow-up CT scan. By then the white area is usually gone or at least smaller. But if it's growing, we perform a needle biopsy or remove it.

In my 1999 *Lancet* study, we found abnormalities on the baseline scans of 233 participants. We expected that the vast majority of these spots would prove to be harmless. Instead of subjecting everyone to the discomfort of a needle biopsy, we used a high-resolution CT scan to examine suspicious growths in more detail and to measure them. Because CT images can be combined by computer software into a three-dimensional picture, we're able to measure tumors much more accurately than is possible with a two-dimensional x-ray.

At first, we relied mainly on size to decide what to do next. If a *nodule* (a small mass) was 11 millimeters or larger (bigger than a small lima bean), we recommended an immediate biopsy, because large nodules have a greater chance of being cancerous. Some smaller nodules were biopsied immediately because their appearance suggested a malignancy. Otherwise, we recommended a follow-up high-resolution CT scan three months later. We compared the second image to the first. Only if the nodule grew at a rate typical for lung cancer did we recommend a biopsy. If the lesion remained the same size, we suggested monitoring it with a repeat CT scan a year later.

Following this plan—which we called the Henschke protocol—we recommended biopsies for only 28 of the 233 people whose initial scans showed areas of concern. All but one of those who underwent biopsies had lung cancer.

By now we've refined our criteria, based on research findings. Because the screening protocol changes as our knowledge increases and technology advances, we post the current updated version online at *http://ICScreen.med.cornell.edu*. If you decide to be tested, I urge you to ask your doctor to check the site so you can be sure your test results are evaluated according to the very latest protocol.

How Often Should You Be Checked?

We recommend annual CT tests for current smokers, a very-high-risk group. We don't yet know how often people at lower risk need to be checked, though we assume it's less frequently than once a year. As more research is completed, we'll have a much clearer picture.

Other Screening Techniques

CT is not the only method under consideration for lung cancer screening. Here are others that hold promise for use alone or in combination with CT or other techniques:

CT Images of the Same Lesion, Three Months Apart

By combining adjacent CT "slices" with computer software, we can create an enlarged three-dimensional image of a nodule and track its growth.

First CT image

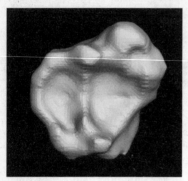

CT image three months later

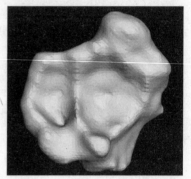

This is the same nodule seen in the CT image on page 49. The nodule is about 7 millimeters in length, about the size of a pea. Because this abnormality might have been a harmless benign lesion, we asked the patient to return in three months for a repeat scan.

This picture shows the same nodule three months later. A benign lesion would have remained unchanged; however, this nodule has grown to 8 millimeters. A biopsy confirmed that it was cancerous, and the nodule was surgically removed. The diagnosis was adenocarcinoma, stage 1A—the very earliest stage of lung cancer. The patient's prognosis is excellent.

Chest X-rays

Chest x-rays are still used to find lung cancer before it becomes symptomatic. Though standard x-rays are not nearly as sensitive as CT scans, screening by chest x-ray is better than no screening at all. Enhancements in x-ray technology can improve lung cancer screening in locations where the spiral CT is not available.

One significant advance is computerized chest x-ray analysis, which

Information for Doctors

For the latest I-ELCAP lung cancer screening protocol, see *http://ICScreen.med.cornell.edu.*

ELCAP's first report appeared in *Lancet* in 1999: "Early Lung Cancer Action Project: Overall Design and Findings from Baseline," C. I. Henschke et al., *Lancet* 1999; 354(9173):99–105.

Since then, more than two dozen articles about lung cancer screening research have been published in medical journals. For a current list—which also includes citations to seminal earlier articles—see *http://www.ielcap.org.*

helps doctors find smaller lesions. A lung x-ray can be confusing to look at. Crisscrossing the picture are front and back ribs. Arteries, veins, and bronchi run through the lungs. Even an experienced radiologist might miss a subtle thickening that signals cancer. With computer assistance, suspicious areas can be highlighted, so the radiologist can examine them with particular care. Nodules usually aren't seen on a standard chest x-ray unless they're at least 30 millimeters (a little over an inch) in diameter. But with computer assistance, lesions as small as 9 millimeters become visible.

Sputum Cytology

Despite the discouraging findings from the 1970s, sputum cytology has enormous potential for lung cancer screening. The technique can find cancers at a very early stage, even before they're visible on CT scans. Its value may be improved by these recent advances:

Sample Collection

One limitation of sputum cytology is the difficulty most people have when they try to cough up an adequate sample of fluid from deep inside their lungs. Thus a negative test result doesn't necessarily mean that someone is

> ## Why Do I Have to Wait?
>
> **Q**UESTION: *I had a CT scan and my doctor found a tiny suspicious area in my lung. She wants me to repeat the CT in three months. But I'd much rather deal with it immediately.*
>
> **ANSWER:** Difficult as it is to wait, that's really the best approach with a very small suspicious area in the lung. Most likely, it's not cancerous. By waiting to see if it grows, your doctor spares you an unnecessary lung biopsy, which is an invasive, uncomfortable procedure.

cancer-free. One promising innovation helps produce a sample by having the person inhale a medication that ordinarily is used to thin the respiratory secretions of people with cystic fibrosis. To be screened, the person puffs on the inhaler, sits for a few minutes to allow the medication to take effect, then coughs. Other sputum production methods under investigation include use of humidifiers to loosen secretions. It has been difficult to find a humidifying method that's both effective and comfortable, but efforts continue.

Markers

Originally, sputum cytology simply involved a search for abnormal cells. However, now we know much more about the very early changes involved in cancer. Researchers are investigating several new kinds of markers—substances found in sputum that could signal cancer or a precancerous condition. For example, investigators at the H. Lee Moffitt Cancer Center and Research Institute in Florida and the National Cancer Institute have reexamined an archive of sputum specimens and clinical data from the old Johns Hopkins study of sputum screening. They selected samples taken from participants who showed no sign of lung cancer at the time, but who later developed the disease. Using the archive, they identified certain mutations in oncogenes and tumor suppressor genes that appeared in sputum cells one to thirteen months before any other evidence of lung cancer.

Test Readings

Other advances hold promise for improving the ease and accuracy of sputum test readings. For example, special dyes can highlight abnormal cells.

As with Pap tests, computer-assisted reading can speed processing and reduce errors in interpretation.

Blood Tests

Some day a simple blood test could screen for lung cancer. Researchers are looking for substances in the blood that could flag the disease. One promising possibility involves evidence of damage to the p53 gene. Damage to this tumor suppressor gene is strongly linked with cancer, including lung cancer. The p53 gene produces a protein, called the p53 protein, that regulates cell growth. When the gene is damaged, the cell produces abnormal p53. The body responds by producing p53 antibodies, which can be detected in the blood. These antibodies are rare in healthy individuals, but are often found in the blood of people with cancer.

Breath Test

A breath test, similar to the one used to identify drunk drivers, might be able to spot people at high risk for lung cancer. A multicenter study published in *Lancet* in 1999 checked the breath of 108 patients who had suspicious chest x-rays and were about to undergo further diagnostic tests. Looking at twenty-two chemicals found in the breath, investigators were able to correctly predict the presence of lung cancer in 72 percent of the cases.

I dream of the day when my insurance company will send me a postcard reminding me to get my annual screening for lung cancer, just as they send me a reminder postcard for my mammogram every year.
—Selma

We know that lung cancer can be cured if it's found early enough. Now—after two decades in which screening was abandoned as hopeless—we're renewing efforts to make it possible. I expect that research will establish the lifesaving potential of screening, that standards will be set, and that costs will fall. We will have taken one giant step toward containing the deadly epidemic of lung cancer.

CHAPTER 6

Are You at Risk?

I was a heavy smoker for over twenty years. During that time I never smoked less than a pack a day; sometimes it was two. Most of my adult life I worked in construction, and was therefore exposed to things like wallboard dust, drywall dust, gypsum, wood resins, pressure-treated lumber, paint fumes, and probably asbestos too. I have a picture in my mind of a day when I was cutting bricks. Red dust was coming up. I wasn't wearing a gas mask. It would have been inconvenient because I had a cigarette hanging out of my mouth.

I couldn't say, "How could this possibly happen?" Still, the diagnosis was a shock. I knew people with similar or even worse lifestyles who didn't develop lung cancer.

—Jim

Anyone can get lung cancer. However, the odds are much higher for some people than for others. Are you at risk? The answer depends in part upon your exposure to carcinogens—cancer-causing chemicals (especially those in tobacco smoke) and radiation. But that's not the whole story. You've probably heard about people who manage to celebrate their hundredth birthday in excellent heath, despite smoking a pack a day. These folks do *not* prove that cigarettes are good for you! But they underscore the fact that risk involves personal vulnerability—for example, your genetic heritage and respiratory health—as well as exposure to carcinogens. This chapter dis-

Alan Landers—The Winston Man

If you read newspapers and magazines in the late 1960s and early 1970s, you probably saw pictures of Alan Landers. Tall, dark, and handsome, he modeled for countless print ads and billboards as the Winston Man. Sometimes he was shown in a tuxedo, looking macho and sophisticated; or he was embracing a beautiful woman in a romantic setting. Occasionally, the pose suggested a happy family gathering. But always, Alan held a cigarette. "I was expected to portray smoking as stylish, pleasurable, and attractive," he says.

Alan began smoking at age 9, shortly after his father died. "My three older brothers said I had to become a man," he recalls, "so I started smoking." His father had smoked; his three older brothers smoked. Men on TV and in the movies smoked—John Wayne, Montgomery Clift. By the time Alan's modeling career began, he was up to two and a half packs a day.

Smoking was part of the job when Alan worked for Winston. He recalls: "They wanted a quarter-inch of ash on the cigarette. So you'd have to light up and take a few drags. The smoke plume had to look appealing. They'd say, 'Blow out more,' or 'That's too much.'" Sometimes Alan puffed through more than a pack of cigarettes to achieve just the right spiral of smoke or length of ash. "By the time you finished a week of shooting," he says, "you could hardly breathe."

Alan continued to smoke after his years as the Winston Man. In 1987 he entered the hospital for a hernia operation—and a preliminary x-ray revealed that he had lung cancer. Today, the former model and actor—and former smoker—has a new career: he lectures on the dangers of tobacco.

To reach Alan Landers, visit his web site (*http://www.winstonman.com*) or call 954-731-3017.

cusses factors in both categories. We'll also tell you about many ways to reduce your lung cancer risk, from limiting exposure to carcinogens to making healthy lifestyle changes.

Smoking

Smoking is by far the most significant cause of lung cancer, accounting for about 85 percent of all cases. Tobacco smoke contains at least fifty-five known carcinogens. Twenty of these—including benzopyrene, chromium, N-nitrosamine, cadmium, nickel, and arsenic—have been linked to lung cancer in animals or humans. Your lung cancer risk is closely correlated with your smoking history.

Estimating Tobacco Exposure

The measure most commonly used to summarize smoking history is the *pack-year*, the equivalent of smoking one pack of cigarettes per day for a year. For instance, if you've been smoking for ten years, and have always smoked two packs a day, your smoking history is 20 pack-years. Most smokers aren't that consistent. So you might need a few minutes to do the calculations. (See example below.)

Estimating Pack-Years: Example

PAT'S SMOKING HISTORY	PACKS	YEARS	PACK-YEARS
Pat started smoking occasionally as a high school junior, averaging about 5 cigarettes (a quarter of a pack) per day.	¼	2	½
In college, Pat smoked more—about a pack a day.	1	4	4
For the next ten years, Pat smoked approximately a pack and a half a day.	1½	10	15
During a stressful period that lasted about three years, Pat's smoking increased to two and a half packs a day.	2½	3	7½
Pat cut back to a pack a day for nearly one year, then quit completely.	1	1	1
Total pack-years of smoking			28

The Dark Truth about Light Cigarettes

"Light" cigarettes are just as harmful as regular ones, despite their lower tar and nicotine numbers. Those measurements are made by special machines that supposedly mimic how people smoke. Light cigarettes have pinpoint holes in their wrappers, which dilute the smoke with fresh air—at least when a machine lights up. But in real life, smokers cover up the tiny holes with their lips or fingers, so they inhale extra tar and nicotine. Also, if a cigarette doesn't supply the nicotine they crave, they compensate by taking more or deeper drags.

Some experts believe that the trend to light cigarettes could explain the recent rise in adenocarcinoma, the form of lung cancer that affects smaller airways and the alveoli (air sacs) deep inside the lungs. Before light cigarettes became popular, squamous cell and small cell lung cancers—which strike the larger airways—were more common.

When researchers want to study people at elevated risk for lung cancer, they usually recruit individuals with a smoking history of at least 10 to 20 pack-years. But smoking behavior is also relevant to risk. Two people with the same pack-year history may not have the same exposure to cigarette carcinogens. For example, one person's exposure may be greater because he or she inhales more deeply and always smokes cigarettes down to the very end, while the other typically puffs lightly and stubs out quickly.

Regardless what or how you smoke, quitting helps. The odds slowly improve with each smoke-free year, though ex-smokers always have a significantly greater risk of developing lung cancer than those who never smoked. In Chapter 7 we'll offer many suggestions to help you quit if you haven't already done so.

Other Kinds of Smoking

Tobacco cigarettes are not the only problem. Other smoked products also carry significant health risks, including lung cancer.

- **Cigars and pipe tobacco** contain the same carcinogenic compounds found in cigarettes. Though cigar and pipe smokers have lower rates of lung cancer than cigarette smokers do, that's because they usually light up less frequently and are less likely to inhale. However, when people accustomed to cigarettes switch to cigars or pipes, they tend to inhale, often without realizing it.

- **Marijuana** produces the same kind of damage to the lungs that cigarette smoke does. That's not surprising: marijuana cigarettes contain more tar than tobacco cigarettes—and they're not filtered. Though marijuana smokers typically consume fewer cigarettes than tobacco smokers do, they inhale deeply and hold the smoke in their lungs.

- **Bidis and kreteks,** exotic flavored cigarettes, are unknown to many adults but alarmingly popular among middle and high school students. Many youngsters believe they're safer than regular cigarettes. Not so. Both are just as addictive and carry all the same health risks, including lung cancer. Bidis, which aren't filtered, are especially dangerous: since they're more loosely packed than typical American cigarettes, the smoker must puff harder and more frequently to keep them lit.

- **Herbal cigarettes,** which are sometimes sold in health food stores, may contain tobacco. Even if they don't, they have similar levels of tar and their smoke contains many of the same kinds of irritants as tobacco cigarettes. Though their health hazards haven't been researched, they can be presumed to carry a risk for lung cancer.

Secondhand Smoke

If you spend time with people who smoke, you're exposed to secondhand smoke—a mix of "mainstream" smoke exhaled by smokers and "sidestream" smoke from burning tobacco. The chemical composition of both kinds of secondhand smoke is similar to what smokers inhale. The Environmental Protection Agency estimates that 3,000 nonsmokers per year develop lung cancer because they're exposed to other people's tobacco smoke at home or at work. The thicker the cloud, the greater the risk.

For information on secondhand smoke and nonsmokers' rights, contact Americans for Nonsmokers' Rights (510-841-3032; *http://www.no-smoke.org*) and Action on Smoking and Health (202-659-4310; *http://ash.org*).

Not the Legacy They Intended

Alice Stewart Trillin, a lifetime nonsmoker, was diagnosed with lung cancer in 1977 at age 38. She couldn't be certain what caused her cancer, but her mother smoked almost three packs of cigarettes a day and her father smoked cigars. Alice commented on her childhood exposure to secondhand smoke in a January 24, 1987, *New York Times* op-ed supporting a ban on public smoking:

> *My parents did everything in their power to insure that I grew up healthy—regular medical and dental checkups, healthy food and orthopedically correct shoes, confinement to the house for what seemed at the time like the entire polio season each summer.*
>
> *I was their only child, my mother almost died giving birth to me, and I'm sure that they would have given up their lives to protect me. They certainly would have given up smoking if they'd had any idea that it might one day harm me. But they had no idea.*

Exposure to Other Carcinogens

Carcinogens are all around us. We can't escape them entirely, but we can nearly always reduce our exposure. That's important because many carcinogens are **synergistic**. In other words, when you're exposed to more than one, their effects don't merely add up—they multiply. Here are the carcinogens most relevant to lung cancer risk:

Radon

The leading cause of lung cancer in nonsmokers is radon—a colorless, odorless radioactive gas that is found in soil. We've known that radon can cause lung cancer ever since the 1930s, when a colleague of Claudia Henschke's father made the connection in Czechoslovakian miners. Miners are still at risk. But we now know that they're not alone. Radon can seep into

Are You Exposed to Radon at Home?

The U.S. Environmental Protection Agency (EPA) estimates that nearly one house out of every fifteen has elevated radon levels. Test your home for radon unless you live on the third floor or above. It's easy to do.

Buy an EPA- or state-certified radon test kit at your local hardware store or from the National Safety Council (800-557-2366; *http://www.nsc.org/ehc/radon/coupon.htm*). The cost is usually $10 to $20. The kit is placed in your basement for a few days, then mailed to a laboratory. Results are returned a few weeks later. A similar long-term test may be needed if the score is high. If you learn that your home has elevated radon levels, you can usually fix the problem inexpensively.

buildings and accumulate in poorly ventilated rooms. If this happens in your home, you could inhale dangerous amounts.

In the lungs, radon releases tiny bursts of radiation that can damage lung tissue and lead to cancer. The risk is much greater for smokers. According to the Environmental Protection Agency (EPA), radon contributes to up to 10,000 lung cancer deaths annually. For more information, contact the EPA's National Radon Hotline (800-SOS-RADON) and request its free booklet called *A Citizen's Guide to Radon*; or read it on the EPA's radon web site (*http://www.epa.gov/iaq/radon*).

Other Radiation Exposure

When radon is inhaled or radiation is directed to the chest, lung cancer risk is increased. If your job requires you to wear a radiation badge, you know you're exposed at work and need to observe safety precautions.

For most of us, the best way to minimize radiation exposure is to avoid unnecessary medical x-rays. However, in many instances, the benefits outweigh the risks. X-rays are valuable tools for diagnosing injuries or illnesses; they're also used for treatment. Fortunately, current techniques have greatly reduced unnecessary radiation exposure to the lungs during cancer therapy. But several studies have found an elevated incidence of lung cancer in breast cancer survivors who received radiation treatments long ago; within this group, the risk is significantly higher for smokers. While long-term survivors need to know about the risk—especially if they smoke—this threat is much less for today's patients.

Asbestos

Asbestos is a mineral that was widely used in construction and manufacturing from the 1940s to the 1970s. When asbestos is crushed, it breaks into tiny fibers. If these fibers are inhaled, they may damage the lungs. The effects usually are seen only decades later.

People exposed to asbestos in their work have a much higher than normal incidence of lung cancer. This includes people involved in asbestos mining and manufacture, as well as those who work with asbestos-containing products such as brakes or insulation. The risk is greatly compounded for individuals who smoke. Nonsmokers exposed to asbestos are ten times more likely to get lung cancer than other nonsmokers—but for smokers with similar asbestos exposure, the risk is *ninety* times higher.

Though asbestos is used much less now than in the past, many older buildings contain asbestos products, such as insulation, shingles, or floor tile. If these are in good condition, they pose no significant risk to occupants. But

Minimizing Your Risks at Work

Your employer has an obligation to inform you of any on-the-job dangers and to protect you from them. Safety standards are set and enforced by the Federal Occupational Safety and Health Administration (OSHA) or through an OSHA-approved state program. Our advice:

- Get acquainted with the risks. For instance, if you're exposed to chemicals, find out what they are and how they might harm you.

- Keep track of the carcinogens you've been exposed to at work, and tell your doctor when you provide a medical history.

- Follow all safety recommendations. Learn what steps to take in case of an accident or other emergency.

Pets at Risk

Animals can get cancer too—including lung cancer. The environmental carcinogens that damage our genes also damage theirs. Veterinary experts estimate that a quarter to a half of pets that live ten years or more will eventually die of cancer.

The symptoms of lung cancer in pets are the same as in people:

- Noisy breathing, coughing, respiration problems

- Reluctance to exercise, lack of stamina

- Unexplained weight loss, loss of appetite

Diagnosis is usually confirmed by x-ray. Treatment—as for humans—can include chemotherapy, radiation, or surgery.

dangers arise if old asbestos deteriorates and begins to crumble, or if dust is raised by renovations or repairs. For more information, read *Indoor Air Pollution Fact Sheet on Asbestos,* available from your local American Lung Association chapter, or visit *http://www.lungusa.org/air/air00_aesbestos.html.*

Other Occupational Hazards

Experts estimate that each year 10,000 to 12,000 Americans develop lung cancer from exposure to carcinogens at work. The culprits include hazardous chemicals, as well as asbestos, radon, radiation, and secondhand smoke. The dangers are particularly great for smokers who are also exposed to these substances.

━━━

I worked for the county government, in an old warehouse that had a smell like rotten eggs. The vents were full of black soot. People were being diagnosed with cancer, one after another.

The county hired someone to do a study. They declared the building perfectly safe and said, "Forget about it." We didn't forget about it. We tracked who got cancer and where they sat. There were about seven hundred people in the building. Over the previous ten years, there had been one cancer diagnosis every three months. I worked in one area where there was a cancer cluster. We later learned that herbicides and pesticides had been stored right above the floor where we were working.

I was diagnosed with lung cancer in 1997. I'm not a scientist, and I can't prove that the building was the cause of my cancer. I was a former smoker, which put me at risk. I loved my work, but I took early retirement because I didn't want to return to that building.
—*Joyce*

Air Pollution

If the air you breathe every day irritates your eyes and makes you cough, it's probably harming your lungs. Chronic exposure to air pollution has been linked to lung cancer, as well as to asthma, chronic bronchitis, and emphysema. For advice on protecting yourself, see *The Inside Story: A Guide to Indoor Air Quality*, a free booklet from the Environmental Protection Agency's Office of Air and Radiation (800-438-4318; *http://www.epa.gov/iaq/pubs/insidest.html*).

Personal Vulnerability

All of us are exposed to carcinogens, but not everyone gets cancer. Here are factors associated with an individual's vulnerability:

Family History

If you have a family history of lung cancer—your parents or siblings have had the disease—you are at higher risk. The association can be explained in part by shared environmental hazards, such as exposure to tobacco smoke and other pollutants in the home. But careful studies that take account of these issues suggest that genetic factors are at work too. Indeed, in specific subgroups of lung cancer patients—including those who develop the disease early and nonsmoking women with adenocarcinoma—

Tally Your Risk Factors

The questions below highlight the most significant risk factors for lung cancer. Note that this is not a scientifically validated questionnaire. And it's definitely not a substitute for lung cancer screening or a medical checkup. But the more boxes you check, the more important it is for you to address the risk factors you can control and to discuss lung cancer screening with your doctor.

Smoking history

Calculate your pack-year history of smoking, including not only tobacco cigarettes but also other smoking, such as cigars, pipes, marijuana, and herbal cigarettes. (See page 62 for instructions.) Check one box for each 10 pack-years. Examples: If your pack-year history is 20 years, check two boxes; if it's about 25 years, check three boxes.

- Up to 10 pack-years ☐
- Another 10 pack-years ☐
- Another 10 pack-years ☐
- Another 10 pack-years ☐
- Another 10 or more pack-years ☐

Exposure to other lung carcinogens

Check all the answers that apply to you.

- I've been exposed to significant amounts of secondhand smoke at home or work. ☐

the association with family history is greater than it is for breast, ovarian, colon, or prostate cancer.

Lung Disease (Including Previous Lung Cancer)

All lung cancer survivors are at risk for a recurrence or for a new lung cancer; we'll discuss this further in Chapter 16. If you've been diagnosed once, consider it urgent to reduce other risk factors as much as possible.

- I've lived in a home with elevated radon levels. ☐
- I've had unusually high radiation exposure at work or from medical procedures. ☐
- I've been exposed to asbestos ☐
- I've lived or worked in an environment with significant air pollution. ☐

Count the number of boxes you've checked above. If you haven't checked any boxes, your exposure to lung carcinogens is low. Otherwise, the more boxes you check, the higher your exposure.

Personal vulnerability

Check all the answers that apply to you:

- My mother has (or had) lung cancer. ☐
- My father has (or had) lung cancer. ☐
- One or more of my siblings have (or had) lung cancer. ☐
- I have had lung cancer. ☐
- I have emphysema or chronic bronchitis. ☐
- I've had tuberculosis, asthma, or another serious lung disease; or I get pneumonia at least once a year. ☐
- I have other signs of lung problems (see pages 27–28). ☐

Count the number of boxes you've checked in the section on personal vulnerability. If you haven't checked any boxes, your vulnerability is low—though you're not immune from lung cancer. Otherwise, the more boxes you check, the higher your vulnerability.

Your risk of lung cancer is also elevated if you have a history of other lung disease or poor pulmonary function (see pages 27–28 for signs of trouble). This isn't surprising. Problems like chronic bronchitis and emphysema are also caused by smoking or air pollution. But these conditions develop more quickly than lung cancer does, so they can serve as a warning. If you've had tuberculosis, you're also at higher risk for lung cancer. That's because tuberculosis can leave parts of the lungs scarred, and cancer may develop in those areas.

Lifestyle Protections

The body's own cancer-fighting power comes only in part from our genetic heritage. Healthy lifestyle choices contribute too.

The Diet Connection

We know from population studies that people who consume a diet low in fat and abundant in fruits and vegetables have low rates of lung cancer. However, we don't yet know why. Scientists are looking at specific nutrients—including beta-carotene, vitamin E, and selenium—that may be responsible for this protective effect, but answers remain elusive. Nevertheless, it's prudent to follow these nutritional guidelines, which are based on

---

The Mystery of Beta-Carotene

Vitamin A helps our body repair damaged cells and fight infection. We get vitamin A from animal foods, such as cheese and eggs. Plants aren't a direct source, but some fruits and vegetables contain beta-carotene, which the body can convert into vitamin A.

Many studies have found reduced lung cancer risk among people who eat lots of foods rich in beta-carotene, such as carrots, sweet potatoes, and spinach. In the 1980s and 1990s, several large projects were undertaken in the United States and elsewhere to determine if beta-carotene supplements could protect people at risk for lung cancer. The results baffled cancer experts: those taking the supplements—particularly current smokers—were actually *more* likely to get lung cancer than those who received a placebo. The differences were so striking that in 1996 the National Cancer Institute halted a major study of beta-carotene supplements involving more than 18,000 participants.

We still don't have a full explanation for these findings. It could also be that the protective effect of dietary beta-carotene comes from some other as-yet-unrecognized component of fruits and vegetables or from a combination of components. Also, the supplements may affect smokers and nonsmokers differently.

What about Stress?

Emotional stress has many adverse physical effects. Studies have shown that stress makes people more vulnerable to viral diseases such as the common cold. However, it's not yet clear that stress has a similar impact on lung cancer. Still, we know that stress weakens the immune system. Also, stress can be a trigger for smoking. So it makes sense to reduce stress—and to improve your coping skills—as much as possible. See Chapter 15 for stress-reducing methods, including a simple breathing technique that exercises respiratory muscles while helping you relax.

recommendations from the American Cancer Society and the National Cancer Institute:

- Consume five or more servings of fruits and vegetables each day. Select produce in a rainbow of colors to assure variety. Since we don't know all the protective nutrients that plants contain, it's best to cover as many bases as possible. For beta-carotene, include at least one yellow, orange, or deep green vegetable.

- Eat other foods from plant sources several times a day, including breads, cereals, grain products, rice, pasta, or beans.

- Limit consumption of meats and other high-fat foods from animal sources.

Benefits of Fitness

Physical activity seems to protect against several types of cancer, including lung cancer. For example, one study followed nearly 14,000 Harvard alumni over sixteen years, from 1977 to 1993. Those who were physically active were less likely to develop lung cancer. The authors estimated that an average of six to eight hours per week of moderate-intensity physical activity—such as walking or climbing stairs—would significantly reduce lung cancer risk. Benefits were seen in smokers, former smokers, and those who had never smoked.

More research is needed to confirm and explain these findings. One possibility is that exercise boosts the immune system, thereby helping to contain cancer at its very earliest stages. Also, exercise generally improves pulmonary function, which might make the lungs less vulnerable to cancer.

If you haven't been physically active, walking is usually a good way to get started. Some suggestions:

- Set a goal that's well within your capability—an effort that won't cause uncomfortable fatigue or breathlessness. Even five or ten minutes a day is a worthwhile goal at the beginning.

- Begin your walk with a warm-up: a few minutes of walking at an easy pace. Then gradually speed up until you're walking briskly enough to raise your breathing and heart rate, but not so fast that you can't talk. When exercise time is over, slow to an easy pace for a few minutes to cool down. Afterward, stretch your arms and legs to prevent sore muscles.

- Each week, add five minutes to your daily walk, if possible. Aim to build your endurance so you can walk a mile. For optimum benefit, continue to increase the distance or pick up your pace.

Unsolved Mysteries

I was diagnosed at age thirty-six. You think that people who get lung cancer are people who've smoked, or they've worked around hazardous chemicals. None of that fit me. I've never smoked. Except for one job I had for a year, where I was around smokers for about an hour a day, I wasn't exposed to passive smoke. No one in my family had cancer. Jon and I even checked our old house for radon, but the levels were below normal. It's so frustrating. I have no idea what I could have done differently.
—Donna P.

Despite all we know about the causes of lung cancer, some cases defy explanation. Each year in the United States about 26,000 people who never smoked are diagnosed; many of them have no known risk factor for the disease. Also baffling are the high rates of lung cancer among women and African-American men.

A Woman's Cancer Now

Until the 1960s, lung cancer was rare in women. But a time bomb was ticking: during the 1940s, increasing numbers of women had taken up smoking. Twenty years later, in the 1960s, the explosive rise of women's lung cancer began. In just three decades, deaths more than quadrupled. In 1987, for the first time, more women died from lung cancer than from breast cancer. Every year since then, the gap has grown wider, as breast cancer fatalities slowly drop while women's lung cancer deaths continue to rise.

Trends in smoking only partly account for this epidemic. Mounting research evidence suggests that women are more vulnerable to tobacco carcinogens than men are. For example, Claudia Henschke's first CT screening project recruited 541 men and 459 women who had no symptoms of lung cancer but who were at high risk. Since there were more men than women in the study, they expected more men among those with lung cancer. In fact, there were almost three times as many women as men. Other studies have reported similar findings.

Women clearly are at higher risk, but why? We have some tantalizing leads, but we won't know the full story until more research has been done. Estrogen appears to play a role. Genetic factors may be involved too. A University of Pittsburgh study put the spotlight on a gene called the gastrin-releasing peptide receptor gene (GRPR), which is more active in women than in men—and which also is linked to abnormal cell growth in the lungs. And a study from the M.D. Anderson Cancer Center suggests that the capacity to repair DNA may be lower in women than in men.

The Unexplained Vulnerability of African-American Men

African-American men have especially high rates of lung cancer. The incidence of the disease is one and a half times higher among black men than it is among white men. Though scientists have struggled to explain this extraordinary discrepancy, the reasons are not fully understood. Adding to the mystery is the fact that African-American women have only very slightly higher lung cancer rates than do their white counterparts.

One explanation is that African-American men are more likely to smoke than white men. Moreover, they're much more likely to smoke mentholated cigarettes. But we're not sure if that's significant. On the one hand, when menthol burns, it produces additional carcinogens. However, some research suggests that menthol doesn't really make much difference. And the smoking patterns of black men aren't different enough to account for the racial gap in lung cancer rates.

Also relevant is the fact that African-American men suffer from greater exposure to air pollution. They're more likely than white men to live in cities, and to hold industrial jobs that involve toxic dusts. Diet could be a factor. African-American men consume more fat and fewer fruits and vegetables than white men, a pattern linked to higher rates of lung cancer. Yet another possibility is that there's some genetic difference that makes for greater vulnerability.

———

I started smoking when I was thirteen. I'm black, and the world in which I became a teenager was a world that encouraged smoking, rewarded smoking. We were the target of cigarette companies on radio ads and billboards everywhere. Smoking was hip. It was something you did to become part of the scene. Your father smoked, all your peers smoked. Everyone smoked in the clubs. All the musicians had cigarettes hanging out of their mouths.
—Glenn

———

Chemoprevention: The Next Step Against Cancer

The hope of chemoprevention is to intervene at cancer's earliest stage, either by preventing genetic mutations or by keeping damaged cells from multiplying. People at high risk could take chemopreventive medication to ward off lung cancer; medication also could be given to lung cancer survivors to prevent recurrence, just as drugs that reduce blood cholesterol or inhibit clotting are given to those at risk for heart attacks. But the quest is challenging. Unlike chemotherapy, chemoprevention is intended for healthy people who show no sign of cancer. Also, chemoprevention must be administered over a long period. Thus even minor side effects and risks are unacceptable.

Leads to chemopreventive agents for lung cancer have come from epidemiological studies. Sifting through data on large populations, scientists search for subgroups with unusually low rates of lung cancer, then look for reasons. Perhaps some characteristics of their diet or lifestyle might explain it. Here are a few of the substances with chemopreventive promise for lung cancer that are currently under investigation:

- **Retinoids**—derivatives of vitamin A—are essential for normal cell differentiation. Animal studies have demonstrated that retinoids can suppress malignancy in cells exposed to carcinogens, and there's evidence that they can reverse very early stages of cancer in humans. Inhaled retinoids have been proposed as a chemopreventive for human lung cancer, but have not yet been proved safe and effective.

- **Vitamin E** is an antioxidant. That means it protects the body against oxidation, a chemical process that damages our cells in the same way that rust corrodes metal. Several epidemiological studies have found an association between high intake of vitamin E in the diet and low lung cancer risk. Food sources of vitamin E include vegetable oils, whole grains, nuts, seeds, and leafy green vegetables.

- **Selenium,** an essential trace mineral, is another antioxidant that appears to have chemopreventive potential for lung cancer. The most common food sources are meats and bread.

Experts estimate that at least a third of all cancer could be prevented by lifestyle changes. The number is even higher for lung cancer, because smoking is such an overwhelmingly important factor in this disease. If you smoke, quitting is the best step you can take to protect yourself. If you never started or have already quit, you can improve your odds further with additional preventive measures. Regardless of your smoking history, other healthful changes are worthwhile. And anyone who is at risk should consider lung cancer screening, just in case.

Recommendations

For everyone:

- If you smoke, do everything possible to quit (see Chapter 7).

- Minimize your exposure to other lung carcinogens.

- Adopt a healthy lifestyle: eat well and stay fit.

- Have your lungs checked during routine medical exams (see Chapter 3).

- Be alert to any changes in lung function (see Chapter 3).

For those at risk:

- Make sure your doctor is aware of your smoking history and all your other risk factors for lung cancer.

- Discuss lung cancer screening with your doctor (see Chapter 5).

- Consider joining a clinical trial studying chemoprevention or early detection (see Chapter 14).

CHAPTER 7

Encouraging News for Smokers

by Peggy McCarthy

Alan Landers, known as the Winston Man during his successful modeling career, was diagnosed with lung cancer in 1987. His doctor scheduled surgery to remove two lobes of his right lung. He warned Alan not to smoke for ten days before the operation. Alan recalls:

> *I promised, but I just wasn't able to stop. The night before my surgery, the doctor caught me smoking in the hospital waiting room. He screamed at me: "How can you smoke when you're about to be operated on for lung cancer? You're insane!" I cried. I said, "I'm sorry, but I can't help it."*

During his difficult recuperation, Alan managed to quit. But a few years later, at a New Year's Eve party, he lit up—and was hooked all over again. He explains:

> *Everyone around me was smoking. Plus, I'd had a martini. I thought I could handle one cigarette, but it doesn't work that way.*

Four and a half years after Alan's first bout with lung cancer, the disease recurred. He endured another operation, this time to remove a lobe of his left lung. Alan was left with just two lobes, one on the left and one on the right. After that, he finally stopped smoking for good. He says:

> *Smoking isn't an option for me—it's suicide. I'm fighting for my life.*

A Personal Note from Peggy McCarthy

I started smoking in 1958. I was in college and nearly everyone in my sorority smoked. My friends offered me cigarettes. Smoking made me feel I was part of the group. Over the next decade, I graduated, married, had two children, and divorced. Along the way, I made several serious efforts to stop. But I'd start again.

In 1967 I was a single mother with two daughters, Susan and Pam, plus a full-time job. One afternoon I was driving the girls home from childcare, smoking as usual, half listening to their prattle and half thinking about what to get for dinner. Susan's second-grade class had just started a unit on the harmful effects of tobacco. Suddenly, her words grabbed my full attention. She said: "If you really loved Pam and me, you'd stop smoking."

When we got home, Susan opened my purse and took out the pack of cigarettes. She marched to the bathroom, where she proceeded to tear up my cigarettes and flush them down the toilet. Pam thought this was great fun. The two girls gleefully retrieved the pack next to my bed, the pack on the coffee table in the living room, and the full carton in the pantry—and down the toilet went all the cigarettes in the house. I didn't intervene. But late that night, desperate for a cigarette, I went to my car, picked a few butts out of the ashtray, and smoked those. On the way to work the next day, I replenished my supply. I wasn't ready to quit.

Susan and Pam continued to make a game of checking my purse and destroying or hiding any cigarettes they found. (Years later, when we moved, I discovered cigarettes behind the refrigerator.) I still smoked at work, but I was finally cutting back at home. Then one morning in 1968 I woke up and somehow knew I would never smoke again—and I haven't for more than thirty years.

No matter how long you've smoked, quitting helps. Even people like Alan, who stop smoking only when they have lung cancer, gain meaningful survival advantages. You'll reap other important health benefits—and you'll improve the odds for everyone who is exposed to your secondhand smoke.

As a former smoker, I know from personal experience how difficult it is to give up cigarettes. But eventually I succeeded—and you can too. This chapter describes fresh approaches and new medications that ease the process. You'll be encouraged to learn that you don't have to suffer, and you don't have to gain weight.

It's Never Too Late!

If you smoke, quitting is by far the best thing you can do to help your lungs and to reduce the likelihood of getting lung cancer or suffering a recurrence.

- **If you have lung cancer:** Your cancer won't disappear—but your prognosis will be much better if you stop smoking now. You'll also reduce the odds that the cancer will return. One study of 611 lung cancer survivors found that the risk of a recurrence was approximately six times greater for those who continued to smoke.

Smoking Accelerates Aging

Kids light up to look older—but most grown-ups aren't so eager to speed the process. Here's how smoking makes you old before your time:

- *Skin wrinkling:* Smokers are more likely to develop premature wrinkles.

- *Impotence:* Middle-aged men who smoke are twice as likely as nonsmokers to experience erectile dysfunction.

- *Earlier menopause:* On average, women who are current smokers go through menopause one to two years earlier than nonsmokers; ex-smokers fall between the two.

- *Osteoporosis:* Smokers suffer more bone loss as they age. This means there is greater risk of stooped-over posture, fractures, and loss of height.

- **If you've been smoking for two decades or more:** Hyperplasia (excess growth) and dysplasia (abnormal growth) may have started in your lungs. If you stop smoking now, new areas of hyperplasia and dysplasia are much less likely to appear, and your immune system might be able to destroy existing precancerous cells.

- **If you've been smoking for a decade:** The cells in your lungs may have suffered genetic damage. But if you quit now, your body's defenses might be able to repair them or to stop precancerous changes.

- **If you just started:** If you can stop quickly, your risk for lung cancer may drop to the level of a nonsmoker's. The younger you are, the more important it is to quit. Smoking does the greatest damage to developing lungs. It's heartbreaking that smoking has penetrated middle schools, and that some kids are starting to smoke as early as age eight or nine.

The Other Health Benefits

According to the Centers for Disease Control and Prevention, more than 400,000 Americans die each year from causes directly related to cigarette smoking. All of these dangers are greatly reduced when you quit.

You know that smoking causes lung cancer. There's more. Tobacco also is linked to cancers of the mouth, throat, esophagus, larynx, pancreas, bladder, kidney, and cervix—as well as to lung metastases from other cancers. Stroke and lethal respiratory diseases are connected to smoking too. But the biggest health risk is heart disease. The incidence is *triple* for smokers.

If you're a mother or a mother-to-be, your children are harmed by your smoking. The ill effects of tobacco begin before birth. Nicotine narrows the blood vessels in the placenta, so the developing baby receives less oxygen and nutrients. Carbon monoxide, along with toxic substances in cigarettes, cross the placenta and enter the baby's bloodstream. Studies consistently show that the babies of nonsmokers are healthier. If you stop smoking, you're less likely to miscarry or have a stillborn baby; your baby is less likely to be born prematurely; and your baby's birth weight is more likely to be normal.

Secondhand smoke is even more damaging to children than to adults. When you quit, you reduce your child's risk of sudden infant death syndrome, ear and respiratory infections, asthma, and other medical problems. You'll also be a better role model: children of nonsmokers are much less likely to become smokers. When I think back to my smoking years, my most painful memory involves car rides with my daughters. In that confined space, second-hand smoke is so concentrated that it's almost as if I'd forced them to smoke.

The Challenge of Nicotine Addiction

Most smokers have tried to stop at least once. Why should it be so difficult? The main reason is that nicotine, a chemical component of cigarette smoke, is addictive.

⎯⎯

From a secret tobacco industry document, written in 1972 and later uncovered by litigation:

> *The cigarette should be conceived not as a product but as a package.*
> *The product is nicotine.*
> —William L. Dunn, Jr., Philip Morris Research Center

⎯⎯

"I'm Not Really a Smoker."

Surveys suggest that occasional "social" smoking is becoming a more common pattern, thanks in part to restrictions against smoking in the workplace, public areas, and private homes. A California survey found that as many as 20 percent of smokers may be in this category: they might smoke when they're at a bar with friends, but they have no trouble abstaining when they're in a "no smoking" environment. Some social smokers get hooked, but others continue to smoke only occasionally.

How hazardous is an occasional cigarette? We really don't know. However, since the dangers are related to exposure, we can assume that occasional smokers have a higher risk of lung cancer and other tobacco-related ills than nonsmokers. And they're also at risk for becoming addicted.

How Nicotine-Dependent Are You?

Take this simple test—called the Fagerstrom Test for Nicotine Dependence—to find out how dependent you are on nicotine. The answer will help you determine which measures can best help you stop smoking. For each question, write the appropriate number of points on the right. Then add up the points and check your score below.

How soon after you wake up do you smoke your first cigarette?
Within 5 minutes (3 points)
6 to 30 minutes (2 points)
31 to 60 minutes (1 point)
Over 60 minutes (0 points)

Do you find it difficult to refrain from smoking in places where it is forbidden (e.g., in church, in a library, or in a movie theater)?
Yes (1 point)
· No (0 points)

Which cigarette would you most hate to give up?
First of the day (1 point)
Any other (0 points)

When you inhale cigarette smoke, nicotine enters your bloodstream rapidly. It reaches your brain in about ten seconds, stimulating the same parts of the brain that cocaine and heroin do. These areas are called "reward pathways" because they regulate feelings of pleasure and well-being. Each puff provides a fresh nicotine hit. New research suggests that these pleasurable reactions may be enhanced by monoamineoxidase, another psychoactive ingredient contained in cigarettes. There's evidence that genetic characteristics may make some people particularly sensitive to these effects.

Over time, smokers also become accustomed to the emotional effects of nicotine. They rely on cigarettes to calm them down, to perk them up, and to help them focus. Smoking, like alcohol, serves as a social lubricant. And it becomes a habitual part of everyday life—breaks at work, the accompaniment to coffee at the end of a meal. On top of all this, nicotine acts like a diet

How many cigarettes do you smoke per day? □

> 10 or fewer (0 points)
> 11 to 20 (1 point)
> 21 to 30 (2 points)
> 31 or more (3 points)

Do you smoke more in the first hours after waking than during the rest of the day? □

> Yes (1 point)
> No (0 points)

Do you smoke even when you are so ill that you are in bed? □

> Yes (1 point)
> No (0 points)

TOTAL POINTS □

NICOTINE DEPENDENCE	SCORE
Low	0 to 3
Medium	4 to 5
High	6 to 10

SOURCE: "The Fagerstrom Test for Nicotine Dependence: A Revision of the Fagerstrom Tolerance Questionnaire," by T. F. Heatherton, L. T. Kozlowski, R. C. Frecker, and K. O. Fagerstrom, in *British Journal of Addiction* 1991; 86:1119–1127. Used with the permission of Karl Fagerstrom.

pill: it suppresses appetite and speeds metabolism. Surveys suggest that as many as 40 percent of female smokers use cigarettes to control their weight. That's why tobacco companies market long, slender cigarettes to women, and give them brand names like Virginia Slims. All of these factors—the physical craving, the emotional and social dependence, the habit, and the fear of weight gain—explain why it's so tough to quit.

> The year before my lung cancer was diagnosed, my doctor told me, "You really should stop smoking."
> I made the decision to quit. I talked to people who had stopped, and asked them how they did it. My best friend said, "It's simple self-control. You'll want a cigarette and you'll just have to say no."

> *I was a carpenter and because I worked for myself, I could control my own schedule. I selected a job site where I'd be alone in the middle of nowhere. I purposely left my cigarette pack at home, went, and did the work. I remember coming home, wanting a cigarette, and saying no, I'll just eat something instead. I had assumed I'd fail. But when I made it through the first day, I realized I could do it.*
> —Jim

The Latest Medical Treatments

The more nicotine-dependent you are, the more likely that cravings, depression, or distressing weight gain have derailed your previous attempts to quit. New medical approaches could make it possible now:

Nicotine Replacement

Nicotine replacement products ease the withdrawal symptoms that you might otherwise experience when you quit. Nicotine is the addictive component of cigarettes. However, the most significant health hazards come from the tar and carbon monoxide. Though nicotine isn't harmless—it can raise blood pressure, speed the heartbeat, and cause heartbeat irregularities—these risks are much smaller than the enormous risks of continuing to smoke. But after you've used a nicotine replacement product to stop smoking, it's very important to systematically decrease your daily dose. The tapering-off process usually takes about ten weeks.

Consider nicotine replacement if your previous attempts to quit ran aground because of withdrawal symptoms, or if you scored "medium" or "high" on the nicotine dependency test. Studies show that these products can double the chances of success.

Nicotine replacement is now available in four forms: patches, gum, nasal spray, and inhaler. New versions—including lozenges and lollipops—may be available soon. Select the method and dose that seem most appropriate. Your doctor or a smoking cessation counselor can advise you; also, read the table on pages 88–89 and review information from product manufacturers. If cravings aren't reduced sufficiently, try a different method or a higher dose.

On the Horizon

Among the promising new approaches to smoking cessation under investigation are:

- **Methoxsalen,** a drug used for severe psoriasis. It blocks an enzyme essential to nicotine metabolism. Normally, blood levels of nicotine rise after smoking, then fall as the body metabolizes the nicotine. When blood levels become low again, the smoker experiences an urge for a cigarette. In an experiment at the University of Toronto, smokers given methoxsalen cut back by about 30 percent even though they'd been told to smoke as usual.

- **Antismoking mouthwash,** a mouthwash that alters the taste of cigarette smoke to make it disagreeable. It is being studied at the School of Dental Medicine at the State University of New York at Buffalo. If it proves effective, this product could be especially valuable for pregnant women and others for whom nicotine replacement is not recommended.

- **Nicotine-blocking vaccine,** which keeps nicotine from entering the brain. It could make cigarettes less appealing to smokers. Research on the experimental vaccine is being supported by the National Institute on Drug Abuse.

A few important cautions:

- Read the warning label. Discuss nicotine replacement with your doctor if you are pregnant or nursing, if you have heart disease or high blood pressure, or if you are taking medication for depression or asthma.

- Follow all directions carefully.

- Never smoke while you're using a nicotine replacement product—the combination could cause you to ingest a dangerous amount of nicotine.

- Remember that nicotine is addictive and harmful in any form. Follow instructions for tapering off replacement products, so you don't substitute a new dependency for cigarettes.

Comparison of
Nicotine Replacement Products

METHOD	ADVANTAGES	DISADVANTAGES
PATCH Looks like an oversize bandage. Applied once a day; slowly releases a steady dose of nicotine that is absorbed through the skin. Available over the counter.	Easy and convenient to use.	Can cause skin irritation. Nicotine reaches the brain slowly (after at least two hours) via the skin. Can cause sleep disturbances if worn overnight, which is necessary to prevent morning cravings.
GUM Chewed briefly, then parked between cheek and gums, releasing nicotine that is absorbed through the lining of the mouth. Available over the counter.	Convenient to use. Flexible dosing that can coincide with cravings. Nicotine reaches the brain in about 10 minutes.	Not appropriate for people with dental problems. Effectiveness depends on compliance with special chewing instructions, which some people find difficult.

Bupropion (Zyban, Wellbutrin)

Bupropion is a prescription antidepressant, sold under the brand name Wellbutrin, which mimics some effects of nicotine on the brain. A version

METHOD	ADVANTAGES	DISADVANTAGES
NASAL SPRAY Sprayed into the nostrils as needed, delivering nicotine via the lining of nasal membranes. Available by prescription.	Convenient to use. Flexible dosing that can coincide with cravings. Nicotine reaches the brain in about 5 minutes—fastest delivery method.	Can irritate the nose and throat; not recommended for those with allergies, asthma, or other respiratory conditions. More likely than other nicotine replacement products to cause dependency.
INHALER Device, resembling a cigarette, that contains a cartridge of nicotine. Puffed nicotine is absorbed by the lining of the mouth. Available by prescription.	Flexible dosing that can coincide with cravings. Nicotine reaches the brain in about 15 minutes. Mimics the habitual hand motions of smoking.	Can cause coughing, throat irritation, and upset stomach. Less convenient to use than other methods, because each dose requires repeated puffing.

containing smaller doses of the same drug is marketed as Zyban and has been approved for smoking cessation by the Food and Drug Administration. Bupropion is highly effective in countering nicotine withdrawal—and you don't have to be depressed to benefit.

Research shows that taking bupropion can double the chances of quitting successfully, compared with going cold turkey. The odds are even better when bupropion is used along with nicotine replacement products. An additional benefit is appetite reduction, which helps prevent weight gain.

Since bupropion takes time to become effective, treatment starts a week before you quit smoking. The most common side effects are insomnia and dry mouth. People with seizure or eating disorders, or those taking other antidepressants, should be sure their doctor knows their full medical history before bupropion is prescribed.

Other Treatments

Many people have found acupuncture and hypnosis useful when they try to quit. (See Chapter 15.) There's no conclusive research evidence that these methods work, but since they're safe they're worth trying if you think they might help.

This Time Can Be Different

Surveys of American smokers find that more than 70 percent have tried to stop at least once. Many succeed. According to the U.S. Centers for Disease Control and Prevention, about half of those who have ever smoked have quit.

Some people are able to give up cigarettes on their first try. But many more go through at least three cycles of stopping and starting before they quit for good. Don't be discouraged if previous attempts haven't worked out. They weren't a waste of time! In the process you gained skills and information that will help you succeed in the future. Some suggestions:

Talk to Your Doctor

Your physician will be delighted to hear that you plan to quit. Here are some questions to raise:

- Ask about the particular health benefits you can expect, as well as the risks you'll avoid by quitting.

- Discuss the pros and cons of nicotine replacement and medication.

- Find out if there are programs in your HMO or in your community that could support your efforts.

Figure Out What Will Work for You

Think about what has helped in the past, and what hasn't. Consider your level of nicotine dependence (see pages 84–85):

- **If your nicotine dependence is low:** You may be able to quit "cold turkey" on your own. If this hasn't worked in the past, add additional behavioral measures, such as a support group.

- **If your nicotine dependence is medium:** Nicotine replacement products may be helpful. If they haven't been sufficient in the past, try a higher dose. Or join a group for additional support.

- **If your nicotine dependence is high:** A combination of measures— nicotine replacement, other medication, and support—gives you the best odds of success.

Ask Your Family and Friends to Help

Don't hesitate to call on others for support—your partner, family, friends, coworkers, neighbors. You don't have to fight this battle alone. For-

Information for Doctors

Despite the enormous risks of smoking, surveys suggest that only half of adult smokers have ever been counseled to stop by their health care provider. Yet a doctor's involvement can have a significant impact. So it's very important for physicians to ask *all* patients—not just those with tobacco-related symptoms—if they smoke, to encourage smokers to quit, and to support their efforts.

The U.S. Department of Health and Human Services offers guidelines for doctors: *Treating Tobacco Use and Dependence* (U.S. Public Health Service, 2000). See *http://www.surgeongeneral.gov/tobacco* or call 800-358-9295.

Avoiding Weight Gain

When you quit smoking, you lose the appetite-suppressing and metabolism-speeding effects of nicotine, as well as the oral gratification. On top of that, food begins to taste better. So it's not surprising that many people gain weight when they give up cigarettes. Though this is one of the most dreaded consequences of quitting, the problem is rarely severe—just a few pounds on average.

Experts warn against attempting to diet while you're trying to quit. It's just too tough to battle food deprivation and nicotine withdrawal simultaneously. After you're a solidly established nonsmoker, you can tackle any extra weight with renewed confidence in your ability to make difficult changes.

In the meantime, a few simple techniques can prevent (or at least minimize) weight gain:

- Consider using bupropion, with or without nicotine replacement.

- Exercise—you'll burn calories and reduce stress.

- Keep healthy low-calorie snacks available for when you're hungry.

- Try to eat slowly and with pleasure.

- Drink plenty of fluids—they help you feel full. But limit caffeinated beverages (which may make you jittery), as well as sugary soft drinks, fruit juice, and alcohol (which pile on calories).

mer smokers are especially helpful, because they've been through the process. Ask everyone for a little extra understanding in case you're distracted and irritable while you make the adjustment.

Phyllis—who quit for good twenty-five years ago—describes her struggle and the all-important role of a close friend when she nearly gave up:

> My son was about to turn thirteen and I asked him what he wanted for his birthday. I was expecting him to request something like a new bicycle or a stereo system. He said, "I want you to stop smoking." My heart dropped. He was asking me to give up my best friend. I loved to smoke. I smoked three packs a day. But I stopped.

Quitting was the hardest thing I've ever done. Five seconds didn't go by that I didn't think of cigarettes. If you smoke three packs a day, you're smoking cigarettes when you're doing everything. When I stopped, I could do nothing. I couldn't drive the car because you needed a cigarette to get it started. I couldn't talk on the phone; I couldn't cook; I couldn't be with people.

About two weeks into it, in the middle of the night, I genuinely thought I was going to die if I didn't have a cigarette. I called my friend Paula. It was two a.m. but she came over with a brown paper bag filled with Life Savers, chewing gum, bouillon cubes, raw vegetables, and cinnamon sticks. She held me while I sobbed and shook and sweated. She made me bouillon, and she stayed with me until I didn't feel I was going to die anymore.

How to Help a Loved One Stop Smoking

Friends can play a major role in helping a smoker to quit. The ideal approach does *not* include hostile confrontation, threats, put-downs, preaching, or nagging—guilt is one more reason to reach for a cigarette.

Try to see the problem from the smoker's point of view: cigarettes help to deal with stress, to relax, to concentrate, and to prevent boredom. It takes a lot of courage to quit. Here are ways to be helpful:

- With your friend's permission, tell other friends and ask for their support.

- Offer a survival kit of carrot sticks, sugarless gum and candy, toothpicks, snacks, pencils, and games.

- Celebrate Quit Day and other landmarks by sending balloons, cards, flowers, etc.

- Visit frequently. Be available.

- Never nag, threaten, or criticize. Offer praise and encouragement.

Adapted with permission from the Canadian Lung Association brochure *I'm a Friend of a Smoker*, available at *http://www.sk.lung.ca/content.cfm/friend*.

Try a Smoking Cessation Program or Support Group

Structure and encouragement can be enormously helpful when you're trying to change behavior. A program or group can walk you through the quitting process, provide many how-to tips, and offer lots of support. Many are inexpensive or even free.

Here's how to locate an appropriate program or group:

- Ask your healthcare provider for a referral.

- Call local chapters of national health groups concerned about smoking—the American Cancer Society, the American Lung Association, the American Heart Association—to find out what they offer and to ask about other local resources.

- Check with local organizations—including your HMO, community health department, hospitals, Y, fitness center, and adult education program. Many provide services to help smokers quit.

- Contact Nicotine Anonymous, a free twelve-step program. Check your telephone book, or call Nicotine Anonymous World Services (415-750-0328). Meetings are listed online: *http://www.nicotine-anonymous.org*.

- If you are pregnant, contact the American Legacy Foundation's Great Start Quitline (866-66-START) or visit its web site (*http://www.american legacy.org*) for free information and support.

- Investigate commercial programs, such as Smokenders (800-828-HELP; *http://www.smokenders.com*). Check your Yellow Pages under "smokers' treatment" for other listings.

For free online support groups—which are available twenty-four hours a day—visit the following sites:

- Freedom from Smoking Online, a program of the American Lung Association (*http://www.lungusa.org/ffs/index.html*)

- Nicotine Anonymous (*http://www.nicotine-anonymous.org*; click on "Meetings")

- Quitnet (*http://www.quitnet.com*)

Residential Treatment

Selma had tried everything—from nicotine replacement, to bupropion, to hypnosis—but she just couldn't give up smoking. In 1995,
she finally was able to quit. Selma describes the program that made
the difference:

> *That spring I'd begun attending Nicotine Anonymous
> meetings once a week, but I was still smoking. I said to the
> woman leading the meeting, "The only way I'm going to do
> this is if I go away somewhere." She said, "There is a place you
> can go." I was happy. But I was also thinking: You mean I
> really have to do this?*
>
> *The place was Caron Family Services in Wernersville,
> Pennsylvania. They offer a one-week program. I started on
> August sixth. When I got there, I put out my last cigarette. It
> was much easier than if I'd been at home. There were ten of
> us, and we were all going through the same thing at the same
> time. We ate all our meals together; we were in therapy
> sessions together in the morning, afternoon, and evening.
> Some of the other people had been addicted to many things,
> including heroin, cocaine, you name it. They said nicotine is
> by far the hardest addiction of them all.*
>
> *The program helped me tremendously. I have not gone
> back to smoking. I still go to Nicotine Anonymous once a
> week—that's my insurance policy.*

Contact the following for more information about residential
treatment:

- Caron Family Services, Wernersville, Pennsylvania (800-678-
2332; *http://www.caron.org*)

- Mayo Clinic Nicotine Dependence Center, Rochester, Minnesota
(800-344-5984; *http://www.mayoclinic.org/ndc-rst/residential.html*)

The Timetable of Benefits

Your body will change for the better after you quit. Some improvements appear almost immediately. Others emerge over months and years.

- **The first day:** Oxygen and carbon monoxide levels in your blood return to normal. Blood pressure and pulse, which tend to be elevated in smokers, are reduced. Your chance of a heart attack begins to decline.

- **The first six months:** Your lung function increases and circulation improves. You should feel better, with less fatigue and shortness of breath.

- **The first year:** Your risk of heart disease has decreased by 50 percent.

- **In the long term:** Over the next decade, your health continues to improve. Eventually, your risk of stroke and heart disease will be similar to that of people who have never smoked. Your chances of getting lung cancer will be significantly reduced from what they would have been if you'd continued to smoke. Remember, though, that you are still at risk. Be alert to symptoms of respiratory problems and discuss screening with your doctor.

Giving up smoking is a significant challenge. If you want to quit, draw upon all the helpful resources you can muster—from medication, to professional help, to friendship, to spiritual strength. You'll need courage to persevere past the initial discomforts, but the long-term benefits are well worth it.

When Lung Cancer Strikes

CHAPTER 8

Diagnosis
and Staging

In 1994, I was experiencing fatigue, but I thought I knew why. I'm an oncology nurse and I was working ten to twelve hours a day; I was on call on weekends. Also, my Mom was ill and I was making frequent trips—two hundred miles each way—to see her. But when I became too exhausted to put one foot in front of the other, I made an appointment with my physician. As I sat in his office, I felt guilty for taking up his time.

After my exam, I was immediately hospitalized for tests. The diagnosis was inoperable adenocarcinoma of the lung. I felt this couldn't be happening to me. I was chair of American Cancer Society Patient Services; I taught cancer detection and prevention to staff and the community. How could I be so ill and not know it? I was not experiencing any of the symptoms I taught people to recognize as signs of lung cancer.

—Donna M.

———

Because lung cancer screening is not yet widespread, the disease usually is discovered only when symptoms appear. Unfortunately, this doesn't happen until the cancer has advanced. And that's not the only problem. Many early symptoms, such as fatigue and shortness of breath, aren't ones we associate with lung cancer. These problems could have many other simple explanations, from pneumonia or minor respiratory illnesses to insufficient sleep or lack of exercise. As a result, people with lung cancer often delay seeing a doctor.

Finding the cancer is just the first part of the diagnosis. Further tests are needed to determine its type and stage. The entire process may take several weeks. This chapter describes what to expect during this stressful period.

Symptoms

There is no single pattern of symptoms that characterizes lung cancer. The first sign could be a problem that points to the respiratory system, such as difficulty breathing or hoarseness. But the disease may reveal itself in ways that seem completely unrelated to the lungs—for instance, with headaches, back pain, or swollen fingertips. That's because symptoms originate from three very different causes:

- Tumor growth in the lungs, which can block airways or press on nerves

- Metastases to distant parts of the body, especially the brain and bones

- Hormones and other substances secreted by lung cancer cells

Symptoms Caused by Tumor Growth in the Lungs and Chest

It's unfortunate that the best-known symptom of lung cancer—coughing up blood—is not one of the first signs of the disease. If it were, perhaps more people would seek medical attention promptly. But the early symptoms are so ordinary, so easily explained by relatively harmless conditions, that they often go unnoticed.

Fatigue or Weakness

When a tumor blocks an airway, the supply of oxygen in the blood may become insufficient. Fatigue and weakness are the body's protective responses: if we move less, we need less oxygen.

Of course, there are many other reasons for these problems. Perhaps you aren't getting enough sleep. Or maybe you have a cold. But if unusual fatigue or weakness persists, see your doctor. Tests might reveal anything from pregnancy, to mild anemia, to more serious conditions like heart disease or lung cancer.

"If You Hear Hoofbeats, Think of Horses Rather Than Zebras."

Most doctors learn this adage in medical school. It's a valuable reminder to rule out the most common problems first when diagnosing a patient. As you learn about the symptoms of lung cancer, you may become alarmed every time you pant or cough! While we hope you'll become more aware of your respiratory health, we don't want to cause unnecessary fear. The symptoms described here could be signs of lung cancer, but they're much more likely to reflect less serious ailments. Similarly, it makes sense for your doctor to investigate the most obvious explanations first.

Breathlessness

Uncomfortable shortness of breath—called **dyspnea** (pronounced DISP-nee-a or disp-NEE-a)—is another sign that something is wrong with your lungs. Breathlessness is a common lung cancer symptom. But it has many other possible causes, such as asthma, respiratory illness, or heart disease.

It's normal to breathe more rapidly when we exert ourselves. As we age—unless we're conscientious about exercise—we may gradually become less fit. Activities that used to be easy, like climbing a flight of stairs, may require more effort. But you should take notice if the deterioration occurs rapidly, or if you're significantly less fit than your contemporaries.

Kathryne, like many other people with lung cancer, realized only after her diagnosis that she'd been experiencing dyspnea for some time:

I was visiting my daughter in Denver and we went to a balloon festival in the mountains. I was having a hard time breathing. I assumed it was the altitude. But my daughter and sister, who live there, thought it was worse than normal. They took me to an emergency room. I was given a chest x-ray, and that's how my lung cancer was found.

After you go through this, you look back and realize you weren't
up to par but you hadn't noticed it. I had slowed down, but it was
nothing that would say I had a big problem.

Repeated Bouts of Pneumonia

A tumor or other obstruction in the airways can cause pneumonia. Fluids that normally move up and out of the lungs are trapped by the obstruction and can become infected. Blockage is not necessarily from a cancerous tumor, and pneumonia has other causes. But if antibiotic treatment doesn't cure it, or if you're suffering repeated bouts of pneumonia—for example, twice in just a few months—further investigation is needed.

Coughing

Coughing is the body's mechanism for clearing irritants and fluids from the airways. The most common causes are respiratory infections, asthma, smoking, allergies, and polluted air. Lung cancer often produces coughing, but not always. Coughing may appear if the tumor is in the central part of the airways, or if the cancer produces fluid. However, people whose cancers affect the outer portions of the lungs—the smaller airways and alveoli (air sacs)—are less likely to experience coughing.

Most people have coughs on occasion. Smokers often have a chronic cough. How can you tell if there's reason for concern? Your own experience is the best guide. Look for a cough that's different from usual or that has these characteristics:

- Lasts two weeks or more

- Seems more severe or produces more phlegm than your usual coughs

- Involves additional symptoms, such as weakness or breathlessness

- Produces blood-streaked sputum (***hemoptysis*** or coughing up blood)

Smokers generally cough more than nonsmokers do. But if you smoke, you have a baseline that's normal for you. Be aware of any change in your usual pattern. Here's what Jim noticed before he was diagnosed with lung cancer:

My wife and I had bought a fixer-upper. I'd always had a smoker's
cough, but after we moved into the house it was distinctly different.
The cough was racking and very hoarse. As soon as I lit a cigarette, I

Do You Have Dyspnea?

Use this 1 to 5 scale, which is similar to scales that doctors use to evaluate dyspnea, to assess your degree of breathlessness.

1: No dyspnea	*I don't become short of breath except during strenuous physical activity.*
2: Slight dyspnea	*I become short of breath during moderate physical activity, such as when I hurry, walk up a hill, or climb a flight of stairs.*
3: Moderate dyspnea	*I must walk more slowly than most other people my age to avoid becoming breathless.*
4: Severe dyspnea	*I can't walk on level ground for more than a few minutes without stopping to catch my breath.*
5: Very severe dyspnea	*I become breathless during everyday activities like getting dressed or undressed; I'm confined to my house because of breathlessness.*

If you aren't sick but have gradually begun to experience slight or moderate dyspnea, you could just be out of shape. Bring the problem to your doctor's attention if any of the following apply:

• You don't see improvement after a few weeks of regular exercise.

• The condition came on suddenly and wasn't associated with an illness.

• You have severe or very severe dyspnea.

would cough. When I lay down to go to sleep at night, the cough would wake up my wife and me. I would sit on the sofa until it subsided. It got to the point where I had to sleep sitting up. I thought I was allergic to something in the new house.

Any unusual cough requires an explanation. Most doctors first try to rule out pneumonia by prescribing antibiotics. That makes sense, because pneumonia is a lot more common than lung cancer. However, if the cough doesn't improve after a course of antibiotics or if it recurs right away, be persistent about having a CT scan and additional tests. If you're at risk for lung cancer, make sure your doctor knows about your smoking history and any other relevant factors.

Hoarseness

Minor infections can produce hoarseness. Be alert to any unusual hoarseness that doesn't go away in a week or two. Lung cancer tumors can cause hoarseness if they're located near the larynx (voice box) or if they press on the nerves associated with the larynx.

Noisy Breathing

A person who is at rest usually breathes silently. Notice any change in the sounds you make when you breathe. New wheezes, grunts, or other noises could indicate extra fluid or an obstruction in the airways.

Pain or Weakness in the Back, Chest, Shoulders, or Arms

Most of us have occasional aches and pains, especially as we get older. Still, persistent unexplained pain or weakness requires investigation. The most likely cause is arthritis or other degenerative changes in the joints, bones, or muscles. But it's also possible that a tumor is pressing against a nerve.

Difficulty Swallowing

If this problem (called *dysphagia*) persists for a week or more, and isn't associated with a respiratory illness, see your doctor. The cause could be an infection, an enlarged thyroid, or even stress or anxiety. But there's also a possibility that a tumor is compressing or blocking the esophagus.

Swelling of the Face and Neck

Cancer that has invaded the mediastinum (the space between the lungs) may press against nearby blood vessels. The vein that returns blood to the heart from the head, neck, chest, and arms—the superior vena cava—runs through the mediastinum. Blockage of this vein produces a collection of symptoms referred to as *superior vena cava syndrome:* swelling of the face and upper body from excess fluid, distended veins in the neck, and rapid breathing. If the problem isn't addressed, severe headache, blurring of vision, and even loss of consciousness can occur.

Lumps Near the Neck

Any unusual lumps around your neck or collarbone should be brought to your doctor's attention. The lumps could be enlarged lymph nodes, which are a possible sign of lung cancer. However, the most likely cause of enlarged

The Tragedy of Misdiagnosis

Misdiagnosis is a common problem with lung cancer—and it can make the difference between life and death. Many people who call ALCASE describe repeated medical visits, sometimes over many weeks or months, before the true cause of their problem is identified. One of those sad and frustrating calls came from Larry, a CPA in his late 40s.

Larry went to his internist because he had a dull pain on the right side of his middle back, near the shoulder blade. He described the problem and commented, "I guess I'm getting too old for basketball." The doctor agreed that he'd probably pulled a muscle, and suggested hot packs.

A month later, Larry returned. The pain hadn't gone away. "You sit in front of a computer all day," the doctor said. "Get up and move around occasionally; change to another chair." Larry started taking hourly exercise breaks at work. He bought a new chair. When that didn't help, he bought a different kind of chair, one used in a kneeling position. The pain persisted. Still convinced the problem was a pulled muscle, the doctor referred him to a physical therapist. But physical therapy didn't help either. The therapist suggested that Larry see an orthopedic surgeon. At his first appointment, an x-ray was taken so the doctor could check his spine—and a tumor was discovered in Larry's lung. This tumor was pressing on a nerve in his back, causing the persistent pain. By the time the correct diagnosis was made, the disease had spread to both lungs and to lymph nodes in his chest. Larry died about a year later.

lymph nodes in this area is an infection in your mouth or throat. Lumps near the neck also could indicate a thyroid problem.

Symptoms Caused by Metastases Outside the Chest

The earliest signs of lung cancer may come not from the lungs but from distant sites to which the disease has spread. When lung cancer metastasizes, it usually travels to the brain, the bones, the liver, or the adrenal glands. The symptoms below have many possible causes. But sometimes they develop because of spreading lung cancer.

Headaches and Other Brain-Related Symptoms

If lung cancer metastasizes to the brain, it can produce severe headaches, blurred vision, confusion, seizures, or changes in personality or mental functioning. These are very serious symptoms that need to be investigated promptly. If cancer is found, its origin must be determined to plan treatment. Cancers can originate in the brain, but brain tumors may be secondary cancers that started elsewhere—including the lungs.

Glenn describes the symptoms that led to his diagnosis:

My daughter saw something in the newspaper and asked me what it meant. I looked at the newspaper. I saw letters and tried to sound them out, but I couldn't make sense of them. My wife heard me. She grabbed the newspaper and said, "Read this." I couldn't. She looked at me in horror. I said, "Take me to the hospital."

Three weeks earlier, Glenn had been at the same hospital for a complete checkup, including a chest x-ray. His lungs hadn't been clear, but the doctor had assumed it was pneumonia and prescribed an antibiotic—after all, Glenn came down with pneumonia about once a year. When Glenn arrived in the emergency room unable to read, the doctors checked his records, found the earlier x-ray—and told him he probably had lung cancer with metastases to the brain. Tests confirmed the diagnosis.

Bone Pain

When cancer spreads to the bones, it may cause an aching pain. Bones that are compromised by encroaching cancer may fracture easily. If cancer reaches the spine, or if the tumor is pressing on a nerve, symptoms can include back pain.

John's lung cancer was discovered during a physical examination for what he and his doctor had assumed was a gallbladder problem:

> *I would get attacks sometimes when I ate. I wouldn't be able to breathe. One day, while this was being investigated, I woke up a little short of breath. I was fifty-three. I figured, I'm no kid. So I paid no attention to it. That week I went to a gastroenterologist. He was feeling the area where I felt pressure during the attacks, just below my ribs on the right side, in the area of my gallbladder. While he was doing that, he hit my rib cage. I went through the roof. I had never felt such pain. It was like I was stabbed.*

Symptoms Caused by Tumor Secretions

Lung cancer may become visible through effects caused by hormones or other substances that the tumors secrete. When that happens, the symptoms are called *paraneoplastic syndromes*—"para" means "along with"; "neoplasm" means "tumor." Symptoms of paraneoplastic syndromes don't necessarily indicate that the disease has spread. Tumor secretions may reach parts of the body where the cancer itself isn't present.

Weight Loss

People with cancer sometimes lose weight even if they're eating normally. This condition, called cancer wasting or *cachexia* (pronounced ka-KEX-see-a), may include lack of appetite. The effects appear to be triggered by substances that the tumor releases into the bloodstream, as well as by immune system responses to the cancer. If you're on a diet, you know why you're losing weight. But unexplained weight loss of ten pounds or more should always be brought to your doctor's attention.

Changes in the Fingertips

Several changes in the fingers are associated with lung cancer, though they could have other causes. The tips of the fingers become wider and puffier; the nails appear more curved from cuticle to tip, as if they were hunchbacked. This is called *digital clubbing.* The reasons for digital clubbing aren't fully clear, but it should be brought to your doctor's attention because it could signal lung or heart disease.

Digital Clubbing

Fingertips are wide and puffy.
Nails appear curved from cuticle
to tip.

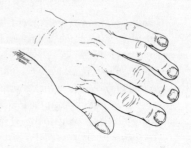

Other Symptoms

Paraneoplastic syndromes (symptoms caused by tumor secretions) can include mental confusion, muscle weakness (especially in the legs), unsteady balance, water retention, night sweats, or hot flashes—all of which can have many other causes. Some signs, such as elevated blood sugar and excess calcium in the blood, often are discovered from abnormal laboratory test results rather than symptoms.

How the Diagnosis Is Made

Lung cancer diagnosis is always a multistep process. Usually it begins with a visit to your primary care provider—the family physician or internist responsible for your overall care. The doctor will take a medical history, perform a physical examination, and give you any tests warranted by your symptoms.

Once lung cancer is suspected, you'll probably be referred to a *pulmonologist,* a doctor who treats disorders of the lungs and chest, or an *oncologist,* a cancer specialist. Additional tests will confirm the diagnosis. If you have lung cancer, your doctors need to learn what type it is and what stage it has reached. You may have some or all of the tests described below, depending on your symptoms and the findings. But the sequence always should be carefully planned to minimize unnecessary invasive procedures.

Review of Your Health History and Current Symptoms

All the doctors you see will ask about your personal and family medical history, as well as your current complaints. Write down your medical history ahead of time (Chapter 10 includes a form to use). Also list your symptoms and any questions you have. *Be sure to mention any relevant risk factors, even if you're not asked about them.* See pages 70–71 to review.

It's surprisingly easy to forget significant information. Estrea, whose unexpected lung cancer diagnosis at age 46 was described in Chapter 1, says:

> I started smoking when I was seventeen and quit at thirty-one. After I quit, I divorced myself psychologically from the whole concept of smoking. I considered myself a nonsmoking person. I'd been going to my internist for ten years, but I don't remember ever mentioning to him that I had smoked.

Physical Examination

During the physical examination, the doctor will investigate your symptoms. If you have respiratory problems or if lung cancer is suspected, the exam will focus on your lungs. The physician will listen to your chest with a

Assemble a Medical File

Begin collecting your medical records as soon as possible. During the days and weeks of your diagnosis, tests may be ordered by different doctors and administered at different facilities. All these records should be sent to each new doctor you consult. But as the papers accumulate—all of them containing important information about you—there's an increasing risk that pieces may go astray. The best way to make sure that your records are complete, and immediately available for any doctor who needs them, is to keep them yourself.

Make photocopies of written reports and test results; ask for copies of all scans. It's much easier to get these records at the time of your tests than it will be to get them later. Medical offices are usually happy to comply with this request. They may charge for the service.

stethoscope and tap your back to detect fluid in your lungs or obstructions in your breathing passages. Since lung cancer may affect many other parts of the body, the doctor may do any or all of the following:

- Check your weight and blood pressure

- Examine your eyes, to see if there are signs of increased pressure from your brain

- Probe the area above your collarbone, checking for enlarged lymph nodes

- Look for signs of fluid retention (*edema*), such as swollen ankles

- Feel your abdomen to see if your liver is enlarged

- Conduct pulmonary function tests, such as spirometry, to check for reduced airflow.

Laboratory Tests

You'll probably receive standard blood and urine tests to check for anemia, infections, or other explanations of your symptoms. If lung cancer is suspected, sputum cytology may be performed. This is a microscopic examination of coughed-up material to see if cancer cells can be found. Unfortunately, it's often difficult to sample mucus from deep inside the lungs. While a positive sputum test can confirm the presence of lung cancer, a negative result doesn't mean that you're cancer-free.

Imaging Tests: Chest X-rays and CT Scans

If your symptoms suggest a problem with your lungs, your doctor may order an x-ray, CT scan, or both. These tests are supervised by a *radiologist*, a physician who performs imaging tests and interprets the results. Make sure the radiologist sees any previous x-rays or CT scans of your chest. If an abnormality has been present for two or more years without growing, it's probably not cancerous.

The same CT equipment used for screening (see Chapter 5) is also used for diagnosis. But there may be other differences. For diagnosis, the machine may be set to a higher resolution so more detail can be seen. Sometimes an injection is given before the scan to heighten the contrast between different types of tissues. Also, a diagnostic CT scan is usually covered by insurance.

> # Why Do I Need a Chest X-ray If I'm Having a CT Scan?
>
> That's a good question to ask your doctor. A chest x-ray may not be necessary if you've had one recently. However, this test is used for many purposes, so it's helpful to have a baseline for future comparisons. For example, chest x-rays are sometimes part of health evaluations before surgery; they may be required by your employer or by an insurance company. Any abnormality requires investigation. In that event, a baseline x-ray would be valuable.

For all these reasons, if you're considering screening, it's important to tell your doctor about any symptoms you're experiencing.

An Important New Test: Positron Emission Tomography (PET)

Positron emission tomography (PET) is an imaging test with the unique ability to point to cancerous sites. PET relies upon the fact that rapidly growing cells—such as cancer cells—gobble up sugar more quickly than other cells. Instead of showing only structures of the body, as x-rays and CT scans do, PET highlights areas where sugar metabolism is particularly rapid. These metabolic hot spots could be cancerous.

The test itself isn't new, but it has a new role in lung cancer. Recent research shows that PET can reduce the need for some of the more invasive procedures used to find metastases and determine the stage of the cancer. A study of 102 people who had been diagnosed with lung cancer found that PET detected metastases in eleven cases where spread of the disease had not been visible by CT and other standard procedures. That's extremely important information. Surgery is not the first treatment if lung cancer has metastasized. The last thing a surgeon wants is to open a patient's chest, preparing to remove a solitary tumor, only to discover that the cancer has spread, so the operation cannot proceed.

At the moment, PET is expensive and not as widely available as spiral CT and x-ray. But this is likely to change quickly. PET scans now have FDA

PET Scan: What It's Like

A PET scan appointment usually lasts from two to four hours. You'll be told to fast before you arrive, so your blood sugar levels are low. (Diabetics receive special instructions.) Before the scan you'll be injected with a small amount of radioactive sugar water. You'll wait about an hour for the sugar to become distributed throughout your body. Then you'll lie on a table that's similar to the one used for CT scans, and your torso will be scanned. That part of the test takes about forty-five minutes. The scan itself doesn't hurt, though it can be uncomfortable to lie still for so long. (Ask if you can bring a pillow and a small personal stereo, which may help.) You'll be able to drive and to resume your usual activities immediately after the test.

approval for determining what stage a lung cancer has reached; Medicare and most private insurers cover them because they're cost-effective as well as easier on the patient. Thanks to portable equipment, which can be shared by small communities, access to PET is increasing. What's more, new equipment can perform both a PET scan and a CT scan simultaneously, providing a diagnosis and information about metastases in less than half an hour.

We urge you to discuss PET with your doctor before agreeing to surgery or other invasive diagnostic or treatment procedures for lung cancer.

Invasive Diagnostic Tests

The following tests allow doctors to perform a *biopsy*—extraction of a small sample of tissue or fluid from suspicious areas inside your lungs for examination under a microscope. A biopsy is necessary to confirm the presence of lung cancer and determine its type. But doctors can't learn from a biopsy what stage the disease has reached.

Because the tests are invasive, we strongly recommend that you have them done by lung cancer specialists if possible. Otherwise, select doctors who have the most experience with the procedure you need. Ideally, they should perform it frequently, not on just one or two patients a month.

Bronchoscopy

A **bronchoscope** is a long, flexible telescope about the width of a pencil, which is equipped with fiber-optic light and a camera. Examination with a bronchoscope, called **bronchoscopy**, allows your doctor to view the inside of your bronchi (the main airways) and to extract samples of tissue and sputum for testing. This test may be recommended if an x-ray or CT scan shows a suspicious area in the central part of your lungs; microscopic examination of the samples can confirm the presence of lung cancer and determine its type. The procedure usually is performed by a surgeon or by a pulmonologist (a lung specialist). One variant is **fluorescent bronchoscopy**, in which the test is performed under a special kind of fluorescent illumination that makes abnormalities more visible.

During bronchoscopy, the bronchoscope is snaked into the major bronchial tubes via your nose or mouth. Sometimes an x-ray is used to help

---

Breast Cancer in the Lung?

Sometimes diagnostic tests reveal that a cancer found in the lungs actually isn't lung cancer. Rather, it's a secondary cancer that has metastasized from another site. Cancers of the breast, colon, thyroid, bone, ovary, testes, or kidney may spread to the lungs. But the type of cancer remains the same, even in the new site. For instance, a breast cancer that metastasizes to the lung is still a breast cancer. Likewise, lung cancer that metastasizes to the brain still looks and behaves like lung cancer, not like brain cancer.

Symptoms of metastatic tumors that come from other sites are similar to those of lung cancer: fatigue, shortness of breath, coughing, and wheezing. But the cells behave differently from lung cancer cells. Proper identification is necessary for effective treatment.

What makes a distant cancer metastasize to the lungs? We don't yet know. However, a study published in *Chest* in 2001 reported that breast cancer is more likely to appear in the lungs if a woman smokes. Further research is needed to learn if the same is true for other secondary cancers that emerge in the lungs.

the doctor guide the tube. To minimize discomfort, you'll be sedated and given local anesthesia. You may also receive medication to suppress coughing and gagging, as well as supplemental oxygen to help prevent feelings of breathlessness. Relaxation techniques (see Chapter 15) can be helpful. The test can take as little as thirty minutes or up to several hours. Expect your throat to be sore for a few days after the procedure.

Fine Needle Aspiration

Another way to obtain tissue samples without major surgery is with *fine needle aspiration*. You'll be given local anesthesia. The doctor—usually a surgeon or a radiologist—will insert a very thin hollow needle between two ribs and into the suspect area, using an x-ray or CT scan for guidance. You may feel brief, sharp pain as the needle penetrates the pleura, the membranes that surround the lung. A sample of tissue will be sucked into the needle. The pathologist can then identify the type of lung cancer, though not the stage.

This procedure is considered quite safe: life-threatening complications are rare and 90 to 95 percent of patients can return home two hours later. However, because of potential side effects—including bleeding inside the lung and lung collapse—it's best for fine needle aspiration to be performed in a hospital. The skill of the doctor is important, especially if the target is very small: it takes considerable expertise to direct the needle to a small area inside the chest.

Extraction of Fluid from Between the Lungs and the Pleura

Fluid sometimes accumulates in the space between the lungs and the membranes that surround them (the pleura). This condition, called *pleural effusion*, can be caused by an infection. But the fluid could be secretions from a lung cancer tumor. Pleural effusion is visible on x-rays and other scans. It can compress the lungs and impair breathing. Fluid may be drained to relieve symptoms, or it may be extracted with a hollow needle to check for the presence of cancerous cells. The extraction procedure is called *thoracentesis*. It's usually performed by a surgeon, radiologist, or pulmonologist.

Tests Performed under General Anesthesia

The following two tests, mediastinoscopy and thoracoscopy, can obtain tissue samples and also examine the inside of the chest. Since either test requires general anesthesia, it's often done just before lung cancer surgery.

Rather than opening the chest immediately after the patient is anesthetized, the surgeon first uses mediastinoscopy or thoracoscopy to make sure the cancer hasn't moved beyond the lung; if it has, surgery is rarely appropriate. The particular test depends on the location of suspected cancer.

Mediastinoscopy (for the Center of Your Chest)

One of the first places that lung cancer spreads is to the lymph nodes in the mediastinum, the space between the two lungs. A mediastinoscopy allows the doctor to view the mediastinum and collect lymph nodes to check for cancer. While you're under general anesthesia, a viewing instrument is inserted through a small incision made just above your *breastbone* (the long, flat bone that runs down the center of your chest). Sometimes one or more instruments are inserted through additional incisions to collect tissue samples or lymph nodes.

Thoracoscopy (for the Periphery of Your Lungs)

Thoracoscopy permits the surgeon to check the lining of your chest and the surface of the lungs for evidence of cancer. A viewing instrument called a *thoracoscope* is inserted through a small incision; other instruments, inserted through additional incisions, can collect tissue samples.

Other Tests to Detect Metastases

When lung cancer spreads, it most often invades the bones, the brain, the liver, and the adrenal glands. Tests to search for metastases include:

- MRI (magnetic resonance imaging) of the brain or bones

- Bone scan

- Ultrasound or CT scans to check the adrenal glands, liver, and bones

Lung Cancer Types, Stages, and Grade

A very important part of your diagnosis is determining what kind of lung cancer you have, what *grade* (how aggressive) it is, and what stage it has reached. This information will guide your treatment.

What Type of Lung Cancer Is It?

Cells from your cancer will be examined under a microscope by a pathologist, a doctor trained to diagnose disease by analyzing fluid and tissue samples. Usually these cells are obtained from a biopsy, though it's sometimes possible to get them from a sputum or pleural fluid sample.

As we explained in Chapter 4, there are two distinct types of lung cancer: small cell (SCLC) and non-small cell (NSCLC). Even before the patholo-

---

Your Pathology Report

Request a copy of your pathology report and add it to your file of medical records. Your doctor can explain any parts that are difficult to understand. Pathology reports include the following:

- Identifying information about you, such as your name and date of birth. Check that the details are correct.

- Description of the tissue samples as they look to the naked eye, without magnification (sometimes called "gross description"). The origin of the tissue—which lung and lobe—will be noted.

- Description of the tissue samples under microscopic examination. This section of the report may be very technical.

- Diagnosis. This is the heart of the pathology report. It describes the type of lung cancer and its stage (if known), any lymph node involvement, and the grade and other characteristics of the tumor cells—for instance, how rapidly they are dividing and whether or not they're sensitive to hormones.

Because the pathology report determines how your cancer will be treated, consider getting a second opinion from a pathologist with special expertise in lung cancer. This doesn't require another biopsy or physical examination; the second pathologist reexamines the same slides. Insurance may cover the cost, especially if the first report was inconclusive or if you have a rare form of lung cancer.

gist's report, your doctors may suspect a particular type of lung cancer because of its location. But confirmation is important for planning treatment and follow-up. Different types tend to grow at different rates and spread to different sites.

What Grade Is the Tumor?

The pathologist will examine cells from the tumor to determine how differentiated they are. Normal cells are differentiated: they have a distinct appearance depending on the function they are expected to perform. The less differentiated the cells, the more abnormal they are and the more aggressive the cancer is likely to be. Tumor cells usually are graded on a scale of 1 to 4, with a higher number reflecting greater abnormality.

What Stage Has the Cancer Reached?

Cancer staging is a standardized way of classifying cancer. You've probably heard people refer to cancer stages; you may know that stage I is early cancer while stage IV is advanced. Staging classifications enable researchers to communicate more clearly and they help doctors plan treatment.

Each type of cancer has its own staging system, but they're all based on the same three factors: the size and invasiveness of the tumor, lymph node involvement, and spread to other parts of the body (metastasis). Small cell lung cancer and non-small cell lung cancer have different patterns of growth and have been staged differently. However, the NSCLC system is increasingly used for SCLC as well.

Non-Small Cell Lung Cancer (NSCLC)

Staging of NSCLC is based on three characteristics:

- **T:** Size and location of the tumor
- **N:** Extent of lymph node involvement
- **M:** Presence or absence of metastases

Non-Small Cell Lung Cancer: T-N-M Classifications

T (Tumor)	N (Lymph Nodes)	M (Metastases)
T0: Cancer cells found in bronchial secretions, but no tumor is visible.	**N0**: No lymph node involvement.	**M0**: No evidence that cancer has spread to other organs or to lymph nodes outside the chest and neck.
T1: Tumor is 3 centimeters or smaller and is completely surrounded by lung tissue.	**N1**: Only lymph nodes within the affected lung are involved; this may include the hilar lymph nodes (nodes near the hilum, the point where the lung attaches to the main airway).	**M1**: Cancer has spread to other organs or to lymph nodes outside the chest and neck.
T2: Tumor is larger than 3 centimeters and is completely surrounded by lung tissue.		
T3: Tumor is any size and has invaded the chest wall.	**N2**: Involvement of lymph nodes in the mediastinum (area between the lungs) on the ipsilateral side (same as the tumor).	
T4: Tumor is any size and has invaded vital structures outside the lung or has produced malignant pleural effusion (fluid between the lungs and the chest wall).	**N3**: Involvement of hilar or mediastinal lymph nodes on the contralateral side (opposite from the tumor).	

The Imperfect Art of Diagnosis

E ven excellent, experienced doctors may miss lung cancer, especially in a person who is at low risk for the disease. Symptoms are not specific to lung cancer and can be misleading. Some tumors, because of their location, are difficult to see on CT or x-ray. Doctors sometimes must revise an early stage diagnosis when previously hidden metastases are found. They may discover that a patient has a different type of lung cancer than previously thought—or actually has more than one kind of lung cancer.

What can you do to minimize diagnostic delays and errors?

• Provide your doctor with complete information about your medical history and relevant risk factors.

• Be persistent if your physician's initial efforts fail to find a satisfactory explanation for your symptoms.

• If you don't respond to treatment as expected, consider the possibility that the diagnosis may not be correct. Seek a second opinion and further opinions if necessary—including a second pathology opinion.

The first step in staging is to assign numerical values to T, N, and M. The higher the number, the more advanced the disease.

The second step in staging is to combine this information into a T-N-M description. For instance, T2-N1-M0 means that the tumor is larger than 3 centimeters and completely surrounded by lung tissue; lymph nodes within the lung are involved; and there is no sign of any spread outside the chest.

Each T-N-M description is associated with a particular stage of NSCLC. (See table on pages 120–121.) For example, T2-N1-M0 is stage IIB.

As you can see, the current staging system assumes that the smallest tumors are about 3 centimeters (equivalent of 30 millimeters) in size. But CT can find tumors of less than 10 millimeters. The NSCLC staging system will be updated as we gain experience with these tiny tumors.

Stages of Non-Small Cell Lung Cancer

STAGE		T-N-M DESCRIPTION	WHAT IT MEANS
0		T0-N0-M0	Cancer cells have been detected in sputum, but no evidence of cancer has been found on chest x-ray or CT. Some of these very early cancers may be eliminated by the immune system. In the future, we may have chemopreventive treatments—medications that can keep these cancers from advancing further.
I	IA IB	T1-N0-M0 T2-N0-M0	Stage I is very early lung cancer that shows no signs of having spread. Chances of a cure are excellent, particularly if the tumor is one of the smaller ones detected by CT. The usual treatment is surgical removal of the affected lobe of the lung. Radiation therapy is used instead when the patient cannot undergo surgery for medical reasons. Chemoprevention and other new techniques—available through clinical trials (see Chapter 14)—may be helpful as well.
II	IIA IIB	T1-N1-M0 T2-N1-M0 T3-N0-M0	Stage II is early lung cancer that has spread to the chest wall or to lymph nodes within the affected lung (including the hilar lymph nodes), but not beyond. Chances of a cure are very good. The usual treatment is surgery to remove the affected part of the lung and the cancerous nodes; sometimes radiation and chemotherapy are administered as well. Radiation alone may be used if the patient is unable to withstand surgery.

STAGE		T-N-M DESCRIPTION	WHAT IT MEANS
III	IIIA	T3-N1-M0 T1-N2-M0 T2-N2-M0 T3-N2-M0	In stage IIIA, the cancer has spread to the chest wall or mediastinal lymph nodes, but it is still confined to the same side as the affected lung. Combinations of surgery, radiation, and chemotherapy offer the best chance for cure or long-term survival. Treatment may begin with surgery; sometimes surgery is delayed until radiation or chemotherapy shrinks the tumor.
	IIIB	T4-N0-M0 T4-N1-M0 T2-N3-M0 T3-N3-M0	In stage IIIB, lung cancer has spread to the opposite side of the chest or is producing malignant pleural effusion. Usually surgery is not recommended. The best hope for long-term survival is a combination of chemotherapy and radiation. Sometimes this treatment shrinks the tumor enough to permit surgery.
IV		M1 with any T and any N	At stage IV, lung cancer has spread outside the chest. Surgery may be possible if both the original tumor in the lung and the metastasized tumor are very small. Though the disease usually is not considered curable at this stage, radiation and chemotherapy—often using combinations of drugs—can do much to extend survival time and improve comfort.

Small Cell Lung Cancer (SCLC)

About 15 to 20 percent of people with lung cancer have the small cell variety. Small cell lung cancer advances more rapidly than non-small cell lung cancer: the cells divide more quickly. Also, SCLC usually involves multiple tumors throughout the lung. These cancers have been categorized as either limited-stage or extensive, though the NSCLC classifications now are sometimes used instead.

Limited-Stage SCLC

Limited-stage SCLC is approximately equivalent to stages I to IIIA of non-small cell lung cancer: one or both lungs and possibly also the mediastinum and lymph nodes in the chest are involved. The usual treatment is chemotherapy and radiation. Sometimes surgery is possible if the disease is found very early and the tumors are located in just one lung.

Extensive SCLC

When SCLC has spread beyond the chest, it's classified as extensive, which is equivalent to stages IIIB and IV. Treatment is usually chemotherapy and radiation.

Throughout this chapter we've described the diagnostic process as if it were a simple journey with a series of stops along the way. In fact, it's more like a roller coaster ride, filled with uncertainty and fear. You may have suspected the worst all along—or you may have been blindsided by your diagnosis. But now you know. The next two chapters will help you move past the shock to take action.

CHAPTER 9

Coping with the News

by Peggy McCarthy

I told the doctor, "You must be mistaken." I told myself that he'd gotten me confused with someone else. In my mind, if you have cancer, especially lung cancer, you're a dead person. I never knew of anyone who survived lung cancer. You'd hear about a movie star who had it, then they died a week later. But I wasn't going to die, so the diagnosis had to be wrong.

—Anita

———

Every time I speak with an ALCASE hotline caller who has just been diagnosed, I'm reminded that it's impossible to know, until it happens to you, what it's like to hear those words: "You have lung cancer." The news may come out of the blue. Or it may arrive after a long series of misdiagnoses and repeated assurances that nothing serious is wrong. In other cases, lung cancer was a clear possibility right from the start.

Regardless of what led up to that moment, I've never talked to a patient who was able to accept the diagnosis initially. Their first reaction was denial:

This can't be happening to me.

How can my doctor be sure it isn't something else?

Denial is a normal reaction to very bad news. It's actually a valuable protective mechanism: by softening the blow, your mind gives you time to adjust.

Expect to experience a wide range of powerful emotions when you learn you have lung cancer: disbelief, a sense of profound loss, anger, guilt—and sheer terror. Just when you need to think clearly so you can make important decisions, your mind may race, making it impossible to concentrate. Sleep may elude you. These are all normal responses to the news that you have a life-threatening illness.

Lung cancer is probably one of the worst personal crises you have ever faced. But you can find the strength to get through it. This chapter is about that early period when you receive the news, share it with the important people in your life, and begin to move forward.

―――

I went to my doctor because I was experiencing shortness of breath and a cough. He listened to my lungs and took an x-ray; afterward, he showed it to me. I could see that one side was very cloudy. He said, "You have fluid in your right lung. I think this is the cause." He pointed to a white spot that was about the size of a dime. I asked, "What do you think it is?" He said, "A tumor."

When you hear the word "tumor," you think cancer. I was terrified. He called the hospital. There were no openings for a CT scan that day, but he insisted, "We need to fit her in." That was even more frightening.

I drove to my husband's office so Jon could come with me. My mind was going a hundred miles an hour. My daughter Jessica was at vacation Bible school, and I was in charge of the car pool that afternoon. I'm telling myself: I have to make sure Jessica and her friends are picked up; I have to stay in control. I'm thinking: I can't have lung cancer.

After the CT, Jon and I went home to wait for the results. When my doctor called, Jon watched my expression, trying to read what he was saying. The doctor told me, "Donna, the CT scan shows many tumors in your lung, and they look to be cancerous." He referred me to a surgeon.

Jon and I couldn't believe it. All those one-word questions were running through our minds: How? Why?

I didn't have time to fall apart. It was about four in the afternoon on the Friday before July Fourth weekend, and I knew the surgeon's office would close at five. When I called, the nurse said, "We have an opening in two weeks." I said, "You don't understand. I just

> ## *"I Need to Talk to Someone Right Now."*
>
> **Y**ou've just learned you have cancer, and have barely begun to absorb the shock. In these first hours after the diagnosis, talking with a sympathetic and knowledgeable—yet neutral—person can be very beneficial. A counselor will answer questions and help you deal with powerful emotions.
>
> Ask your doctor to refer you to a counselor who has experience working with cancer survivors. Or call one of these free support hotlines:
>
> - ALCASE (Alliance for Lung Cancer Advocacy, Support, and Education): 800-298-2436 between 8 a.m. and 5 p.m. Pacific time, Monday to Friday. ALCASE can provide information and support specific for lung cancer.
>
> - Cancer Care: 800-813-HOPE between 9 a.m. and 7 p.m. Eastern time, Monday through Thursday; 9 a.m. to 5 p.m. Eastern time on Friday. Cancer Care's hotline, which is staffed by oncology social workers, deals with people who have all types of cancer.

found out I have cancer." I started crying. She gave me an appointment for the following Wednesday. I got off the phone and then I lost it. I cried and cried and cried.
—Donna P.

Mobilizing Your Emotional Strength

The first days and weeks after a lung cancer diagnosis will be very difficult. People cope in many different ways. Your approach is as individual as you are. But here are a few suggestions, based on what I've learned from people with lung cancer:

Give Yourself Time to Adjust

Your life changes drastically with a lung cancer diagnosis. You'll enter a new world of doctors and hospitals, where you'll learn more than you ever wanted to know about cancer and its treatment. Your closest relationships will be affected. Everyday routines will be disrupted. You may feel that you've become a different person. Even if your prognosis is excellent, you will experience strong feelings of loss and grief. All this is a lot to absorb. Allow yourself time to deal with your emotions. You can nearly always take a few days—or even a few weeks—to get more information, obtain second opinions, make decisions, and prepare for treatment.

John woke up after diagnostic surgery to learn that he had lung cancer and that a lobe of his right lung had been removed. His doctors recommended radiation treatment followed by chemotherapy. John agreed. But first, he went to the Dominican Republic for two weeks. He explains:

> *Friends were getting married, and I'd been planning this trip for over a year. I was weak from surgery, but I wasn't going to miss it. My doctors weren't happy about the delay. But they had been talking to me about quality of life. I said, "Here's quality of life: a fat white guy at the beach instead of a fat white guy throwing up in a bucket."*
>
> *I had a wonderful vacation. We were at a lovely beach club on the Caribbean; the weather was perfect. I was with very special people who knew what I was going through.*

Cultivate an Attitude of Realistic Optimism

As a cancer patient, you'll hear a lot about survival statistics. Remember that these numbers are based on groups of people. But you are a unique individual. The statistics don't cover all the factors that could be acting in your favor. Lung cancer treatment is improving all the time, which means longer survival times even for people with advanced disease.

———

> *The pulmonologist showed me x-rays of a weird, shapeless mass the size of my fist dangling ominously in my lower left lung. The diagnosis: inoperable lung cancer.*
>
> *For days I was incommunicado. I remember the darkness, the absoluteness of the silence in my house. Wishing to secure the future of*

*my dog, I went to a supportive colleague who had dogs like mine. He
told me not to make assumptions, to think positively. Then he told me
his cancer story. He had survived melanoma. That evening I called
my real estate agent, thinking I would die and leave him in the middle
of a transaction. He told me his cancer survival story. The hospital
social worker told me her husband's cancer story: a year earlier he had
completed a clinical trial; so far so good. She told me about her aunt,
who had come out of a hospice to live another twenty-four years. My
depression went away. I got my focus back and my determination.*
—*Carolyn*

Address the Issues You Can Influence

On top of everything else you're coping with, it's distressing to feel that
your life is out of control. An ALCASE caller once said, "I feel like I've been
plunged into a made-for-TV movie, but they forgot to give me my lines." As
soon as you begin to take charge again, you'll regain a sense of mastery. In
Chapter 10 we'll offer many suggestions.

Sharing the Diagnosis

You're reeling from the diagnosis—and now you must deliver painful information to others and cope with their reactions. Like you, they will experience
strong emotions, including fear, loss, guilt, and anger. They may feel helpless,
because they want so much to help you and don't know how.

Think about the kind of response you need. Your family and closest
friends should know that you have cancer. But you don't have to tell everyone
at once. Not everyone is capable of playing a positive role. When people feel
vulnerable and frightened, their reactions may be self-centered or negative.
This can be devastating when you're expecting—and desperately need—loving
support. ALCASE callers sometimes weep as they describe a cousin who greets
the news with a flippant "Well, I told you to quit smoking," or a friend who
interrupts with a lengthy story about her ex-neighbor who had lung cancer.

I suggest you begin with a loved one who will respond in a helpful way.
We all need different things at a time of crisis. Comfort may be found in

someone who simply listens without making lots of suggestions—or in a person who takes charge. You know best what would be helpful.

Consider calling a hotline or speaking with a counselor before you attempt to tell the people close to you. Your own reactions may surprise you the first time you say those emotionally charged words: "I have lung cancer." If you rehearse with an outsider, it may be easier to tell family and friends in the way you want.

How to Break the News

Sharing your diagnosis raises different issues, depending on who is involved—your partner, children, parents, friends, employer, or colleagues. I'll have specific recommendations in a moment. But first, here are some general suggestions:

- Try to arrange for an appropriate setting. Ideal is a quiet and comfortable place where you can sit and talk face to face without distractions or interruptions. If you must use the telephone to inform someone close to you, it's best to select a time when he or she is not likely to be rushed or distracted. For example, if you're calling a person who has young children, wait until after the youngsters' bedtime. Before you start, ask if this is a good time to talk.

- Consider if another person could help you convey the information. For instance, you might want your doctor to talk to family members. If you're delivering the news by telephone to a loved one who will be very upset—say, you're calling an elderly parent who lives in another part of the country—try to arrange for someone else to be there for support when your call comes.

- Begin by warning your loved one that you have bad news, then quickly and briefly explain. Most people need time to digest bad news; they can't absorb too much at once. Watch for signals that they want to hear more, such as asking questions. Several conversations may be needed to convey the information fully.

Spouse or Partner

Your spouse or partner—someone whose life is entwined with yours—is usually the person (other than yourself) most affected by your cancer. He or she will be deeply concerned about you. But be aware that a partner also faces daunting personal issues too: frightening questions about your future together; worry about the new responsibilities entailed in supporting your struggles with lung cancer. (We'll have more to say about caregiving in Chapter 18.) All this requires time to understand and accept.

The pulmonary doctor looked at my x-ray and said there could be a tumor. It was the first time anyone used that word. He gave me a bronchoscopy. You're awake, with a tube up your nose and down into your chest, and they snip pieces of what they think is the tumor. He said, "I saw it—you've got a mass the size of a golf ball." Then he started speaking Greek. I said, "My wife is waiting outside. What do I tell her?" He said, "Tell her you have lung cancer."

Afterward, I tried to be a brave soldier for my wife. I said it was fine. But I was poleaxed. When we were five feet from the car, I started crying.

—Jim

Children

It's natural for parents to want to shelter their children—including adult children—from distressing news. But lung cancer is not easy to keep secret. Even very young children notice when their parents are upset or ill; they may overhear conversations or telephone calls. Normal family activities may be disrupted. If no explanations are provided, children are left to imagine the worst. Sometimes bewildered youngsters assume that they're to blame for whatever is happening. They worry that their other parent will become ill and die, or that they too will succumb to cancer. Teenagers and young adults may feel excluded and unsettled. So it's best to tell your children as soon as possible. Here are some recommendations:

- Gear information to the age of the child. The younger the child, the simpler your explanations should be.

- Encourage questions—but don't provide more information than your child is ready to hear. A good approach is to answer questions briefly and wait to see if your child asks more questions. If not, that's probably because the youngster isn't yet emotionally ready to hear the answer. Sometimes it's helpful to read a book together. There are many wonderful children's books on cancer. See the resource box below or ask a children's librarian to guide you.

• Present information truthfully, but as reassuringly as possible. What if the prognosis is bleak and a young child asks, "Is Mommy going to die?" You could say, "We hope not, but at this point we don't know. The doctor is doing everything possible to help Mommy get better." This is a time to draw on your family's religious beliefs for reassurance.

• Anticipate children's concerns about the impact your illness will have on them. This is true even for children who are grown and living on

Resources for Parents

The following organizations have excellent free brochures and other materials on talking to children about cancer:

• The American Cancer Society offers brochures and online information for parents: 800-ACS-2345 or search online at *http://www.cancer.org.*

• Cancer Information Service of the National Cancer Institute, *Taking Time: Support for People with Cancer and the People Who Care About Them.* Available in brochure form by calling 800-4-CANCER (800-422-6237) or online at *http://www.cancer.gov/cancerinfo/takingtime.*

• CancerBACUP (British Association of Cancer United Patients), *What Do I Tell the Children? A Guide for a Parent with Cancer.* Available online at *http://www.cancerbacup.org.uk/info/talk-children.htm.*

• Centering Corporation sells a remarkably extensive collection of books for children and others facing loss—including cancer. For a catalog, call 402-553-1200, or view the list of books and order online (*http://www.centering.org*).

their own. Explain any new family routines—for example, tell young-sters if a relative will be helping out while you're in the hospital or hav-ing chemotherapy. Try not to be hurt if a child seems more concerned about himself or herself at first than about you.

- Tell your children's teachers or guidance counselors what's happening. Often children's behavior changes in school when a parent becomes ill. Their grades may drop, or they may become troublemakers for the first time. It's important for the staff to understand the underlying cause.

- Arrange for children—including teens and young adults—to talk with other adults. Youngsters may be reluctant to burden you with their feel-ings and questions. Let them know they can talk to their other parent, close friends and relatives, teachers, and others.

- Ask children for their support, and figure out ways they can be helpful. The older the child, the more significant this assistance can be. But even small children can make meaningful contributions. Some family-friendly treatment centers welcome youngsters to chemotherapy ses-sions and arrange for the child to be a helper.

———

Jessica was in fifth grade when I was diagnosed, and they were studying lung cancer. All her friends were coming up to her in school and asking, "Jessica, is your mom going to die?" We told her that yes, I could die—but we also reminded her that her grandmother had cancer, and many other people she knows have had cancer, and they're all alive today.
—*Donna P.*

———

Relatives and Friends

If you have children of your own, you can imagine how you'd feel if they developed cancer or any other life-threatening illness. Your parents may experience similarly powerful fear and sadness. Their reactions will depend on your relationship with them, and on their personalities and personal cir-cumstances. If you are a caregiver to your parents, their responses may be similar to what you'd expect from a dependent child.

―――

I'd been in an automobile accident in February; I'd been diagnosed with lung cancer and had surgery on both lungs in March. In May, I went to my grandson's bar mitzvah in Florida. I had not yet told my mother, who was in her mid-eighties, but I knew I had to tell her then. I put on makeup and I looked terrific. I told my mother I'd had an accident, which she brushed off. Then I told her I had cancer. She said, "Don't say that word." I said, "Mama, I have lung cancer, but I'm fine." I showed her the scar. She looked at it, then looked away. Tears welled in her eyes. She said, "Don't tell anyone in my building. They would talk about Edith's daughter who was going to die. You can tell them about your accident."
—*Anita*

―――

Some people prefer to keep the news within a small circle; others don't mind if casual acquaintances know. The decision about whom to tell is a very personal one. It's your choice whom to include or exclude.

―――

It's difficult for friends and family to express their real feelings about cancer. One dear friend said, "I know you'll get better." That was the last thing I wanted to hear. I wanted her to say that she was scared, that she cared, and that she didn't know what to say.
—*Phil*

―――

Employers and Colleagues

Your employers and colleagues may provide valuable emotional support and practical assistance. But even in a caring environment, your boss and coworkers will be concerned about the impact your cancer will have on your performance. And an estimated 25 percent of cancer survivors experience discrimination at work.

What you disclose will depend on several factors, including your assessment of probable reactions and how much your disease and treatment are likely to disrupt your functioning. Be aware that it would take planning and effort to keep the diagnosis secret. Your physician would need to know that the information is confidential; you would have to explain absences and changes in your appearance—otherwise, your coworkers might speculate and raise questions.

Unless you plan to tell no one at work about your diagnosis, let your direct supervisor know first. It would be awkward if that person found out through the grapevine and felt that you were not being honest about the situation. We'll have other suggestions concerning employment issues in Chapter 19.

―――

I didn't tell people in my professional life that I had cancer. I'm an independent film and video producer and I was concerned that if word went out, I wouldn't be able to get work. I knew I might lose my hair, so I told everyone I was thinking about shaving my head. Then one day I walked in with no hair. Everyone said, "You look great!" They didn't notice I had no eyebrows.
　　—*Glenn*

―――

Unexpected Reactions

When you tell those close to you that you have lung cancer, you understandably expect an outpouring of supportive reactions—love, concern, sympathy, compassion, and offers of help. Your loved ones may provide all this and more. But sometimes people don't respond the way you had hoped.

Brian—with whom I spoke several times on the ALCASE hotline—was diagnosed with advanced lung cancer at age 53. He'd gone to the doctor complaining of wheezing and breathlessness; a chest x-ray revealed tumors in both lungs. Brian hadn't asked his wife to come with him to the appointment, so he was alone when the doctor delivered the devastating news. When he came home late that afternoon, he asked his wife, their 14-year-old daughter, and their 17-year-old son to join him in the living room; their third child was away at college. As Brian told me later:

I told them we needed to talk, that I had serious news. We sat down and I said, "I have lung cancer." No one said a word. I told them about the x-ray; I said I'd be having more tests, and that probably I'd begin chemotherapy in a couple of weeks. I stopped and waited for them to say something or ask questions. The first words out of my wife's mouth were: "Will Robbie have to quit college?"

Brian was devastated. Instead of focusing on the threat to his life, his wife's first thought was about the impact on their children. His son and daughter chimed in, wondering if they'd have to get jobs after school. Even-

How to Respond When Someone Tells You: "I Have Lung Cancer."

It's a terribly painful, difficult moment. You're shocked and afraid, so your instinctive reaction may be to protect yourself. But at the same time, you want to help. Anyone would feel uncomfortable and inadequate. Here are some suggestions:

- Realize and accept your limitations. Your impulse is to say something consoling or to fix the problem. But you can't—there are no magic words for that.

- Express your love or friendship, and offer support. Touch and hug if appropriate.

- Listen. Allow your loved one or friend to express feelings and describe what's happening, even if this makes you uncomfortable. *Don't interrupt with anecdotes about other people or about your own experiences.*

- Exercise appropriate restraint. Don't press for more information than the person wishes to share. Refrain from making accusations—this is not the time to mention that you've been telling him or her to quit smoking for years. Be very cautious about offering unsolicited advice.

- Offer concrete assistance. Perhaps you could drive your friend to medical appointments. Maybe the family needs help with shopping, fixing meals, laundry, or chauffeuring kids. If many people have offered to help, perhaps you could serve as coordinator. Talk to family members too. Suggest that everyone think about what's needed. Wait a few days and ask again. Or send a note renewing your offer, with a list of tasks you could do.

tually they expressed their concern about him and became more supportive, but Brian remained hurt. Later, a therapist explained to him that their reaction, though selfish, was normal. At that first horrified moment, his wife and children weren't ready to think about the possibility of his death. So they reached for something more tangible—money—and tried to deal with that.

Here are some ways to deal with disappointing reactions:

- Keep your expectations reasonable.

- Try to think about the situation from their point of view. Of course, that's very difficult when you feel overwhelmed by what's happening to you.

- Be patient. Give them time to cope with the news.

- Talk about fears, to get them out in the open.

- Find support elsewhere—for yourself and for family members. Don't place the full responsibility on those who love you.

I was diagnosed in February. The following Memorial Day, my three roommates from college came from the East Coast to Seattle for a fun weekend. We'd been roommates for four years, back in the 1960s. They rented a gold Cadillac. We drove around, did some sightseeing, went to Mount Rainier, talked, and laughed.
—Ben

Finding Support

We hope that all the important people in your life will be there for you. Many cancer survivors also lean on three other sources of emotional support: individual counseling, patient groups, and their faith or spirituality.

Individual Counseling

When you're dealing with a life-threatening illness, talking to an experienced person—someone caring, but not emotionally involved—can be of great help. Cancer patients receive individual counseling from many sources, including psychotherapists, social workers, and religious or spiritual advisers.

Lisa has a devoted husband, and many good friends. Nevertheless, she says:

> *I couldn't have made it without my psychiatrist. People don't know what to say to you. Every time you talk to your husband, he gets upset—it's hard for someone who loves you to have a conversation about the possibility of your dropping dead. My psychiatrist is a professional, so I can talk to her about whatever is on my mind without worrying about upsetting her.*

Patient Support Groups

Support groups can help ease the emotional burden of cancer; they're valuable sources of information and encouragement. Some insurance plans and HMOs cover the cost of support groups when there's a charge. And many groups are free.

> *I joined a cancer group through the hospital. I'm not a touchy-feely person, but I found the group helpful. It was interesting to compare treatments and doctors, and to see how people were coping. Some were dying and there were tough situations, but it wasn't discouraging. I met people who were very courageous and at peace with themselves. I was inspired to see how they handled it.*
> —Ben

You'll probably benefit from any well-run, supportive group of cancer survivors. However, I recommend finding a lung cancer support group if at all possible (see box on next page). Treatment impairs everyday functioning for most cancer patients. But the impact is more severe when the disease and treatment affect the lungs. For example, lung cancer patients generally experience more fatigue from chemotherapy and radiation than other cancer patients do. Surgery usually is more traumatic for lung cancer patients too: procedures are more invasive and lung tissue is removed, so recovery takes longer. In addition, people with lung cancer may face special issues of stigma and guilt.

How to Find a Support Group

If you are interested in joining a support group, ask your doctor or a hospital social worker to recommend one, or contact one of the organizations below. Also helpful are online support groups. Unlike in-person groups, they're available all the time and require no travel.

- ALCASE (800-298-2436; *http://www.alcase.org*) maintains a list of support groups for people with lung cancer. The organization also has a program called Phone Buddies, which connects patients and caregivers with cancer survivors and family members who are willing to offer support via telephone.

- Cancer Care (800-813-HOPE; *http://www.cancercare.org*) offers support groups for people with cancer and their caregivers. In-person groups meet in New York, New Jersey, and Connecticut. In addition, CancerCare hosts support groups that meet via telephone or online. All CancerCare support groups are free and are facilitated by oncology social workers.

- The Wellness Community (888-793-WELL; *http://www.thewellnesscommunity.org*) provides support for people with cancer at their sites in more than a dozen states.

- Your local chapter of the American Cancer Society (check your telephone book) might be able to suggest a group in your area.

- ACOR (Association of Cancer Online Resources) offers about 100 free online groups, including several focused on lung cancer (*http://www.acor.org*).

- Members of America Online can access AOL's cancer message boards, including one for lung cancer. (Use keyword "Cancer" and select "Lung cancer" from the menu of related subjects.)

- CompuServe's Cancer Forum has a section for cancers of the lung, neck, and head (*http://www.compuserve.com*; follow menus to the Cancer Forum). Non-members can participate.

Participating in a support group doesn't necessarily involve face-to-face meetings. ALCASE's Phone Buddy program offers connections to fellow cancer survivors and their families via telephone or e-mail. Many lung cancer patients benefit from online support too.

Remember that support groups vary considerably, depending on the members as well as on the leaders and sponsoring organization. If you think you might benefit from a group but are disappointed by the first meeting you attend, don't give up! Look for a group that better suits you.

Faith and Spirituality

A cancer diagnosis is a powerful reminder of our limits and our mortality. It brings up issues about life and meaning that many of us usually don't take time to think about. Why are we here? What's truly important? Many cancer patients find strength and comfort in their religious faith as they confront these questions. Others follow a nonreligious path in their search for spiritual answers.

———

The prayers of my family and friends, and my own prayers, are my sustaining factor. Some of the questions will never be answered: Why me? Well, it is me, so let's get through this.
—Donna P.

———

As you face the challenge of lung cancer, you will need to draw on your inner strength and creativity, on your faith, and on your loved ones. In the process you may discover resources you never knew you had. Strange as it may sound, this can be a surprisingly positive experience. Indeed, I've met many people who have come to view this illness, terrible as it is, as the greatest gift they've ever received.

PART V

Taking Charge of Treatment

CHAPTER 10

Preparing for Effective Treatment

The doctor told me, "You've got an inoperable tumor in your left lung. You need to get your affairs in order." The world swirled around my head. My wife was wailing. I asked, "Why is it inoperable?" He explained it was too close to the mediastinum, and there was evidence of spread to the lymph nodes.

I saw another doctor and he said, "There's a study from Memorial Sloan-Kettering. They shrink the tumor with chemotherapy, and it becomes operable. It may be appropriate in your case." He told me he couldn't predict how long I would live. He said, "Chemotherapy is not much fun. And the surgery is rough. But if there's a hope for a cure, it would be from surgery."

I got privileges to read in the medical library. I'd walk into appointments with a list of questions. My doctors were very helpful in explaining things. I came to believe that the best thing I could hope for was to reduce the tumor and then remove it. So I said yes to chemotherapy.

After three rounds of chemotherapy I had surgery to remove my left lung. Though there was no evidence of lymph node involvement, earlier tests had indicated the possibility of microscopic spread. Therefore, I opted for an additional three rounds of chemotherapy. After that I was considered disease-free.

—Jim

Many doctors, even cancer specialists, are not aware of the latest developments in lung cancer treatment. Every day the ALCASE hotline receives calls from people with lung cancer who have been told—incorrectly—that nothing can be done for them. We also hear from patients who have been offered outmoded, less effective therapies. That's why it's essential for you to play an active role in your own care. This means educating yourself, assembling an excellent medical team, obtaining second opinions, and learning to work with your doctors. In a sense, you become the CEO of your disease. No one wants this job. But the effort could save your life. At the very least, it may spare you significant pain and disability. This chapter will help you get started.

Educating Yourself

Lung cancer patients have different management styles, just as CEOs do. Some, the hands-on managers, want to learn as much as possible and to make decisions about their care. Others would rather leave all this to their doctors. Or they might prefer to have a friend or family member act as chief of staff, sorting through the information and guiding them.

Only you can decide which approach is right for you. But we believe that all people with lung cancer should learn the basics. One way is to read this book. Even easier is to read at least one authoritative short brochure or booklet about lung cancer. Your doctor may provide one. Or select one of those listed below; they're all free and easily obtained by calling a toll-free number or visiting a web site. In less than an hour you can master the essential facts. After that, you're ready for more if you wish.

Learning about your disease could change the course of your treatment. Even if you don't discover anything new, information will make the illness and treatment less stressful in some ways. You'll know what to expect, and you'll understand what your doctors are saying.

Basic Brochures and More

No matter how much (or how little) you want to learn about lung cancer, these resources are valuable:

- **ALCASE** (800-298-2436; *http://www.alcase.org*). Telephone counselors can answer your questions and suggest reading material. If you simply want a brief overview, ask for ALCASE's booklet *About Lung Cancer*. For more in-depth information, request the *Lung Cancer Manual*. Or visit the ALCASE web site to download these materials and others.

- **National Cancer Institute's Cancer Information Service** (800-4-CAN-CER; *http://www.cancer.gov/cancerinformation*). Request the informative general brochure *What You Need to Know About Lung Cancer* (or read online at *http://cancer.gov/cancerinfo/wyntk/lung*). You can also obtain helpful brochures on cancer treatment and coping. NCI maintains a comprehensive cancer database, the Physician's Data Query (PDQ), a valuable resource for additional information. The PDQ treatment summaries (one for small cell lung cancer, one for non-small cell lung cancer) review accepted options by type and stage of the disease. The database includes directories of physicians and hospitals, as well as information about clinical trials.

- **Cancer Care** (800-813-HOPE; *http://www.cancercare.org*). Request educational material about lung cancer if you'd like a brief overview. Also ask about teleconference educational programs. The Cancer Care web site has an informative special section about lung cancer, as well as special sections on cancer in the workplace, pain, and other issues of interest.

- **Lungcancer.org** (877-646-LUNG; *http://www.lungcancer.org*), cosponsored by the Oncology Nursing Society and Cancer Care, provides information and support. You can e-mail questions via the web site and a certified oncology nurse will respond within forty-eight hours.

- **American Cancer Society** (800-ACS-2345; *http://www.cancer.org*). Ask for materials about lung cancer. You can also obtain general information on coping with cancer, clinical trials, complementary medicine, and other cancer-related subjects.

Researching Lung Cancer on the Internet

Many valuable information sources are online. If you don't have Internet access at home, you may be able to use a computer at a library or community center. Some hospitals and cancer clinics have patient education

Should I Use a Commercial Cancer Research Service?

Maybe. Commercial cancer research services promise to search medical sources on your behalf and to send you a written report. The typical cost for a search on your cancer is $200 to $500. You might receive helpful information that would have taken you days to compile. On the other hand, the report may be incomplete, biased toward unproven and unconventional remedies, or irrelevant to your situation.

We suggest you start with the free resources listed in this chapter. After you've read these introductory materials, you may feel capable of performing your own research. ALCASE may be able to review the medical literature for you; your doctor can request a PDQ (Physician's Data Query) search on your behalf from the National Cancer Institute.

If you are considering a particular service, try to get a referral from an expert—perhaps your doctor or someone from a patient advocacy group—who is familiar with the service and has seen its reports. Also ask the service if you can see a sample report or speak with a client who has lung cancer.

Whether you do research on your own, receive assistance from ALCASE or PDQ, or purchase a commercial report, discuss new information with your doctor. You may need to arrange a special appointment for this consultation, since it could be time-consuming. Provide a copy of the information at least a week in advance so the doctor can review it prior to your meeting.

areas that include computers. Or you can ask an Internet-savvy friend to find information for you. Print out whatever information seems promising. You will want to read it carefully and discuss it with your doctor.

Even if you're an experienced Internet surfer, you may feel overwhelmed by the amount of information available. Here's a simple strategy for getting started:

- Visit the ALCASE site (*http://www.alcase.org*), Lungcancer.org (*http://www.lungcancer.org*), or another site mentioned above. Read the general information about lung cancer to get oriented.

- Browse through the well-organized and helpfully annotated links at *http://www.lungcanceronline.org*. This superb site was created by Karen Parles, a librarian who is a lung cancer survivor.

For additional information visit these two patient-oriented sites, which cover cancer generally:

- To learn more about researching your disease, check Steve Dunn's Cancer Guide: *http://www.cancerguide.org*. Steve Dunn is a cancer survivor whose site provides intelligent advice about finding information online.

- The National Coalition for Cancer Survivorship has an excellent guide to online resources on cancer, complete with links that will familiarize you with key sources of information: *http://www.canceradvocacy.org*.

These sites are a good beginning; most of them link to many other sites. You'll find additional Internet resources listed throughout this book. Also, ask your doctor for suggestions, and find out if your hospital or cancer center has a web site with information for patients.

It takes time to become familiar with online resources, just as it does to learn your way around a conventional library. But things really do get easier very quickly! Use the features of your browser to record the addresses of useful sites as you explore, so you can locate them again.

A warning: Not all the information you find will be useful—or trustworthy. Anyone can put up a web site; no one polices the content. As with printed materials, keep the source in mind as you read. These articles offer tips for evaluating information you obtain online:

- National Cancer Institute's guide, "10 Things to Know about Evaluating Medical Resources on the Web" (*http://nccam.nih.gov/health/webresources*)

- AARP's article, "Evaluating Health Information on the Internet: How Good Are Your Sources?" (*http://www.aarp.org/confacts.health/wwwhealth.html*)

Finding the Right Doctors

Because medical knowledge advances rapidly, you need doctors who keep up with the latest information—not just one doctor but a team. Usually it's best to be under the care of lung cancer specialists rather than physicians who treat all lung diseases or all cancers.

Consider the hospital as well as the doctors. Leading medical institutions attract excellent physicians and have the most up-to-date equipment and procedures. We'll explain below how to locate top cancer centers. Treatment logistics are simpler if all your doctors are affiliated with the same hospital.

Last, but certainly not least, look for doctors with whom you can communicate and who share your treatment goals. You need not only medical expertise from your doctor but also compassion and encouragement.

The neurologist came into the room. He was a very quiet man. He treated me with respect and he smiled a lot. I was panicked and said, "I have lung cancer and I'm going to die." He said, "That's if you do nothing. But you're going to do something." This was my first moment of hope.
—Glenn

The Vital Importance of a Team Approach

Youthful at age 72 despite stage IV lung cancer, Jules relished travel and a successful postretirement career as a wildlife photographer. But he couldn't help thinking how different his prognosis might have been. Said Jules:

> *Everything depends on the doctor you see. If it turns out that you're going to the wrong physician—one who doesn't know as much, or who doesn't care as much—you're in trouble. That's what happened to me.*

Two and a half years before his diagnosis, Jules had a chest x-ray to check out a persistent cough. The radiologist's report, which was sent to Jules's primary care physician, pointed to an area in the upper lobe of his right lung that was hidden by the rib cage. The report suggested that Jules have a CT scan to investigate further. But his doctor never mentioned the

A Special Kind of Nurse

Your doctors will plan and monitor your treatment. But the oncology nurses will actually be present as you undergo chemotherapy or radiation. They will answer your questions and watch your progress. Because of their training and experience, they are particularly knowledgeable about day-to-day coping with lung cancer.

You can recognize oncology nurses by the initials OCN (Oncology Certified Nurse) or AOCN (Advanced Oncology Certified Nurse) after their names. This means that they have received special training in treating cancer patients, have passed a test, and are committed to continuing their professional education. Certification must be renewed every four years, and nurses are retested every eight years.

suggestion and never followed up. What if the tumor had been found then, before it mushroomed to 6.5 centimeters? What if the surgeon who later removed the upper lobe of his right lung had recommended chemotherapy before and after the operation? Might this aggressive treatment have prevented the metastases to his brain and spine that were discovered six months after surgery? Jules recalled:

> The doctor who diagnosed me referred me to a friend of his, who was a pulmonologist (lung specialist), not an oncologist (cancer specialist). I was in such shock, I was willing to be led, and that was unfortunate. Later, at an ALCASE conference, I met oncologists who specialized in lung cancer. I had never thought about it, but that's whom anyone who has lung cancer should be seeing. If you have heart trouble you see a cardiologist. Most people go to see a general oncologist who treats all cancers. How could that person keep up with all of these cancers?

The first doctor you see—usually your primary care physician or a pulmonologist—may tell you that surgery is indicated or that the only possible treatment is radiation or chemotherapy. This might be correct. But don't make treatment decisions until you have consulted oncologists (doctors who treat cancer) from all three specialties: surgery (surgical oncologist), radiation (radiation oncologist), and chemotherapy (medical oncologist). Specialists' viewpoints differ because they have different training and expertise. For example, a superb surgeon may not know about all the latest advances in chemotherapy or radiation therapy. Often the most effective treatment involves not just one of these approaches but two or three used together. This is called *multi-modality* or *combined modality treatment*.

Getting Referrals

We'd all like to receive our medical care from the very best doctors. But it may take considerable effort to find them. Also, choices may be limited by practical considerations, including money and the constraints of insurance companies or HMOs. (We'll offer suggestions for dealing with medical insurance and managed care in Chapter 19.) Your location also may restrict options. Nevertheless, the most common obstacle is lack of awareness and knowledge—and that's an obstacle you can overcome.

Here are some strategies for locating excellent doctors:

- Ask your own doctor or the physician who diagnosed your lung cancer to refer you to specialists.

- Contact the National Institutes of Health for a referral to the nearest Comprehensive Cancer Center (800-4-CANCER or *http://www.nci.nih.gov/cancercenters/description.html*). The cancer center can refer you to one of its doctors.

Are You Eligible for a Study?

Before you start treatment, investigate clinical research opportunities (see Chapter 14 for more information) or at least raise the question with your doctors. Some studies are open only to patients who are *treatment-naive*—that is, they haven't yet had surgery, chemotherapy, or radiation therapy. Others accept patients only if they've recently undergone a particular treatment such as surgery. So you need to plan ahead if you want to participate.

What If the Doctor You Want Is Not Accepting New Patients?

Doctors, like other professionals, must limit their practices to match their available time. Otherwise they wouldn't be able to give each patient adequate attention. Here are a few suggestions if it's difficult to get a desired appointment:

- Write to the doctor, explaining why you want to see him or her. Mention any unusual features of your case that might make it particularly interesting to the doctor.

- Ask someone else, such as your personal physician or one of the doctor's colleagues, to make the contact on your behalf.

- If an appointment is impossible, ask the doctor or an assistant to suggest another doctor with a similar approach whom you could see instead.

- Request referrals from the National Comprehensive Cancer Network (888-909-6226 or *http://www.nccn.org*).

- Contact the Association of Community Cancer Centers (301-984-9496 or *http://www.accc-cancer.org/members/map.html*).

- See Lung Cancer Online's page of links for finding the best care (*http://www.lungcanceronline.org/care/index.html*).

- Check a well-researched "best doctor" or "best hospitals" article in a local or national magazine. The ALCASE web site (*http://www.alcase.org*) has links to a few such articles of interest to people with lung cancer.

Preliminary Questions

Here are some questions to ask the doctor's office assistant before you make an appointment:

- What is the doctor's specialty? Is the doctor board-certified in that specialty? (See box below.)

- Is lung cancer a special interest of the doctor's? If not, how frequently does the doctor treat patients with lung cancer?

- With which hospitals or treatment centers is the doctor affiliated?

- What insurance does the doctor accept? If the appointment is not covered by insurance, what will be the fee for the consultation and what does that include?

Your First Appointment

At the beginning, you'll probably have basic questions:

- What type of lung cancer do I have?

- What is the stage of my disease?

- What are my treatment options, and which do you recommend?

- What is the goal of my treatment? To cure my disease—or to slow down its progression and to keep me as comfortable as possible?

What Is Board Certification?

Specialists are doctors who have undergone not only four years of medical school but at least three years of supervised training in their specialty and, in some cases, subspecialty. Doctors who have received this additional training must pass a rigorous examination and meet other standards to become certified by one of the twenty-four organizations recognized by the American Board of Medical Specialties (ABMS) and the American Medical Association.

You can verify the certification of a doctor via the ABMS Certification Verification Line (866-ASK-ABMS; *http://www.abms.org*). Its publication *The Official American Board of Medical Specialties (ABMS) Directory of Board Certified Medical Specialists*, which is revised annually, is available in many public libraries.

Lung Cancer and Fertility

In the past, fertility wasn't a common concern of lung cancer patients: the disease typically struck late in life and the prognosis was poor. But it is becoming more relevant now. Smoking starts sooner and lung cancer can be found earlier. Many men and women are delaying parenthood. Also, lung cancer survival rates are improving.

If maintaining fertility is important to you, discuss your concerns with your doctor before treatment begins. Chemotherapy may damage reproductive cells, but certain agents are more harmful than others. For men, options include sperm banking. Women may be able to freeze and preserve ovarian tissue, eggs, or fertilized eggs. If you hope to do this, talk to fertility experts who can advise you about the latest and most successful procedures.

During treatment, potentially fertile couples are advised to use birth control, since cancer treatment—including surgery (and anesthesia), radiation, and chemotherapy—could harm a developing baby. In the rare event that lung cancer is discovered when a pregnancy is already underway, it may be possible to plan treatment so that the pregnancy can continue safely.

As you talk to the physician, you'll learn if this is someone to whom you can comfortably relate. Here are some subjects you may wish to discuss:

- How you can best communicate with the doctor if you have questions or concerns between visits

- The role you wish to play in making decisions about treatment, and the roles that you want friends and family members to play

- Anything about your personal life that's relevant to treatment, such as your job, family obligations, or financial constraints

- Your interest, if any, in participating in research studies or trying experimental treatments

- Your views concerning complementary approaches, such as acupuncture or vitamin therapy

I told my doctor, "These are my needs: I need to be kept on the same page as you're on. I need to know what you're thinking all the time. I can't make decisions unless I have all the proper information."
—John

Do You Need a Second Opinion?

After your diagnosis, your doctors will explain their treatment plan. Should you go ahead, or should you get a second opinion? We believe that an additional opinion is always a good idea (except in the rare cases where severe symptoms require emergency treatment), even if your doctors are renowned specialists at a famous hospital. But under the following circumstances, a second opinion is urgently needed:

- If no treatment is offered. Even if your disease is too advanced to be cured, treatment might be able to prolong your life significantly and make you more comfortable.

Sending Your Medical Records to New Doctors

Most medical offices are very busy and they don't always transfer information promptly. But you won't get the most out of your appointment if the new doctor doesn't have your records. Don't leave anything to chance. Check to make sure that information has been received. Always keep copies of your own records so you can provide them if necessary. Deliver records yourself or use a service that allows you to trace it, such as FedEx or U.S. Postal Service Express Mail. Call the doctor's office beforehand to get the appropriate address for this kind of mailing; call again on the delivery date to make sure the materials arrived.

- If the prognosis is very poor. A second opinion might offer more hope. Or it may simply provide greater clarity, which could guard against later concerns that you or your family didn't do everything possible.

- If your situation is not typical. Each person is unique, and the staging system doesn't take all relevant factors into account. Your range of options may be wider (or narrower) than usual for the stage and type of disease.

- If you're receiving care from doctors who are not specialists. Major cancer centers can provide not only second opinions but also ongoing telephone and e-mail collaboration with your own doctors. This is an excellent option if you live in a small town.

- If you're considering an experimental treatment.

- If you have any doubts about the suggested treatment plan.

Whom to Ask

If possible, seek a second opinion from a lung cancer specialist at a leading cancer treatment center—even if that means you have to travel to a distant location for the consultation. (In Chapter 19 we'll tell you about programs that can help with travel expenses.) Some centers have second opinion programs in which your case is reviewed by a team of specialists, called a **tumor board**.

The purpose of a second opinion is to explore options that your own doctor may not have considered. Therefore, an independent view is best. That usually means seeing someone who is not a close associate of your doctor, preferably a physician who trained at a different hospital and works at a different institution.

When I was diagnosed, I had one brain metastasis. My doctor wanted me to have whole brain radiation. They offer you what they have, and this doctor's facility had whole brain radiation. A neurologist told me to get a second opinion from a separate institution. The other doctor told me I didn't have to have whole brain radiation. He told me about Gamma Knife surgery. The radiation would zap just one spot in my brain, the tumor. I opted for that.
—Glenn

Making Arrangements

Here's how to arrange for a second opinion:

- Talk with your insurance company or HMO. Because this could be a matter of life and death, we suggest that you consider getting a second opinion even if your medical plan doesn't cover it.

- Talk to your doctor. Some patients are needlessly concerned that their doctor might be offended by their wish to consult someone else. On the contrary, physicians usually are pleased to receive additional input. Indeed, your doctor may make the suggestion before you do, or your insurance company may require it. Second opinions are a routine part of medical care. If a physician discourages you from getting a second opinion, consider that a red flag.

- Make an appointment with the physician you wish to consult. To use your time well, prepare a list of questions for the doctor. Have your questions, medical history, and all relevant test results delivered a few days before your appointment so they're available for the doctor to review. (See box on page 152 for delivery suggestions.)

What If the Doctors Disagree?

It's frightening and frustrating for a patient to be caught in the middle when doctors don't agree on the best treatment. Jules, whom you met earlier in this chapter, described his maddening search for answers:

I went for my postsurgical checkup. The surgeon said, "Everything is fine. Go home and enjoy your life." I asked her for a referral to an oncologist; she said I didn't need to see an oncologist. I got a recommendation from someone else and saw an oncologist. He said there was no evidence that chemotherapy was necessary, that he'd give me a chest x-ray every three months.

I saw a magazine article about the country's best oncologists, including one in Florida where I live. I waited five weeks for an appointment. That doctor also said no chemotherapy.

I went to an ALCASE seminar in Washington, D.C., and met oncologists who specialize in lung cancer. I brought my reports. Several doctors told me that if you don't take chemotherapy before and after, you don't have a fighting chance. That put me into a quandary. I went to see yet another oncologist back in Florida. He said there was no evidence that chemotherapy would help me.

When you get these conflicting opinions and time is passing by, you don't know what the hell to do. I got the names of the foremost lung cancer oncologists in the country, and I called them. These were highly qualified doctors—and their opinions were not the same. I was confused; I did nothing.

I'd had the operation in July. The following January I went to a local lung cancer oncologist. I was feeling fine. He took an MRI of my brain, a CT scan of my chest and abdomen, and a bone scan. Everything was not fine. I had a tumor in my brain and a tumor in my spine.

Jules—who died two years after the brain and bone metastases were discovered—believed that chemotherapy before and after surgery would have saved his life. Of course, it's impossible to be certain; nor can anyone know if chemotherapy might have compromised his health instead of improving it.

Here are a few suggestions if your doctors disagree:

- Ask each of them to explain the reasons for his or her recommendations. If possible, arrange for the doctors to speak with each other, to see if their views can be reconciled.

- Discuss the opinions with your primary care physician or another trusted doctor, who may be able to help you sort things out.

- Get a third (or even a fourth or fifth) opinion.

Realize that you may have to make decisions without satisfactory information. In many situations, as was true for Jules, there really isn't a single clear answer.

Working with Your Team of Health Care Providers

Your first weeks as a cancer patient are like a CEO's early days on the job. You'll meet many new people; you'll be bombarded with new information

How Much Time Do I Have to Decide?

You can't know for sure. However, the size of the tumor provides some guidance. If the cancer seems to be less than 1 centimeter (10 millimeters) in diameter, you can probably take a month or even longer to consider your options. If the tumor is larger, you need to decide more quickly. Waiting is always a gamble because some tumors metastasize while they're still very small. Nevertheless, you can nearly always take a few days to several weeks to select doctors and make treatment decisions. If the first doctor you see insists that you start treatment immediately, make sure there's a very good medical reason.

and new responsibilities. All this can become overwhelming. As you begin working with your medical team, adopt routines to manage information and tasks. You'll feel more confident and less stressed when you don't have to worry about forgetting things, and you'll function more effectively.

Establish the Relationship You Want with Your Doctors

Usually one of your doctors will have a central role in your care. You can't always find the ideal match for your personality. But you and your doctors can forge good working relationships. Tracy describes her growing rapport with her oncologist:

> My oncologist works in a small town. He wasn't used to people like me who show up with a list of questions and who want a copy of their file. Over time, he realized that I wasn't questioning his competence but wanted to be treated as a partner in the process. I'd bring him articles. We'd talk about my options. He'd go to a conference and then pass on information to me. It took us a while, but we've gotten a lot more comfortable with each other.

Part of your responsibility as a patient is to communicate effectively with your doctors. Some patients interpret that to mean that they should avoid saying anything negative. In their eagerness to be agreeable, they may say, "Everything is fine," rather than reporting symptoms and asking questions. But you'll be unhappy with your treatment if you withhold information. Don't hesitate to speak frankly with your doctors.

———

Some doctors have a way of not looking at you. If you passed them in the hall, they wouldn't know who you were. I got annoyed with one doctor who was like that. I told him, "This is the face of a lung cancer patient, not the cells in a petri dish. Speak to this face."
—Anita

———

Summarize Your Medical Information

Write one-page summaries of your medications and your medical history. This is information that you will need to provide repeatedly as you meet with new doctors. Use the forms on pages 161–163, or create your own. If you prepare forms on a word processor, it will be easy to update the information and make copies. While you're creating the summary pages, make an emergency card for your wallet.

WALLET CARD	
Name:	Date of birth:
Address:	Phone:
Hospital:	Patient ID:
Insurance company:	Insurance ID:
Allergies:	
Primary care physician (name, phone):	
Primary oncologist (name, phone):	
Emergency contact 1 (name, phone):	
Emergency contact 2 (name, phone):	
All drugs taken currently:	

━━━

I developed a cancer résumé. I write down the basic facts, including the chronology of events and the kinds of treatment I've had. When you've been treated for three years, there's a lot to cover. I use this when I see a new doctor.
—*Tracy*

━━━

Other approaches:

• Use the record-keeping forms in *The Cancer Patient's Workbook: Everything You Need to Stay Organized and Informed,* by Joanie Willis (Dorling Kindersley Publishing, 2001). The book contains extensive additional information for people with cancer.

• Use *The Savard Health Record,* by Marie Savard, M.D. (Time-Life Books, 2000), which has detailed instructions and forms for keeping full medical records, as well as explanations of common medical tests.

• If you don't have time to create a written record of your medications, put all of them in a shoebox or shopping bag and bring them to your first appointment. This is particularly helpful if you're using herbal preparations or supplements that might not be familiar to your doctor.

Keep a Diary of Medical Visits

If your doctor dictates notes after your visit, ask to have a copy sent to you—this is a good way of keeping track of your care. Otherwise, take your own notes or use an audio recorder during visits. Keep all pertinent information: test results, medication doses and instructions, and any other directions. You'll find it difficult to remember everything you're told. It's also hard to recall the names of all the people involved with your care, so write those down too. Between appointments, use the diary to jot down anything you want to discuss with your doctor on your next visit. Send your list of questions to the doctor's assistant a few days before your appointment.

Bring a Friend or Relative to Medical Appointments

Emotional support is always welcome, but a friend or family member can do more. Another person can take notes, fill in missing information, and make sure your questions get answered. If you tend to be shy about voicing complaints or concerns, try to have someone serve as your advocate.

——

A friend drove me to the doctor and she came in with me. I kept saying, "I can do it by myself." But she said, "You'll need someone." She was right. I was unable to focus on what the doctor was saying.
—Anita

——

Get Organized

Even if you've never used a portable calendar and to-do list, these tools will be helpful now. You'll be making many more medical appointments than usual, and will have more tasks to keep track of.

Don't Forget to Mention . . .

Be sure to include the following sometimes forgotten items when you list the medications you take:

- Over-the-counter (nonprescription) drugs that you use regularly, including painkillers, laxatives, antacids, allergy or cold medications, sedatives, and baby aspirin (sometimes taken by adults to prevent heart disease)

- Vitamins, including individual vitamins, "once-a-day" preparations containing multiple vitamins, and vitamin-enriched foods (such as breakfast cereals or meal replacement bars) eaten regularly

- Nutritional supplements

- Herbal preparations

- Birth control pills

- Hormone replacement therapy

- Medicated creams, such as estrogen creams

Keep all your medical information in a distinctive tote bag or briefcase, so you don't forget anything you'll need at your appointments. Also include small comforts or conveniences that could be handy at the doctor's office, such as a book to read while you wait; a cell phone; a roll of coins for the parking meter, vending machine, or telephone; a blow-up pillow if you might want to nap; and a water bottle.

During the weeks after a lung cancer diagnosis you'll make key decisions about your doctors and about your treatment. At the beginning, the task may seem overwhelming. But many resources are available to help. Use them. Within a surprisingly short time you will develop the expertise you need.

Current Medical Information

Date updated:

Name: Date of birth:

Address:

Phone: Fax: E-mail:

Hospital: Patient ID:

Insurance company: Insurance ID:

Allergies:

Pharmacy (name; phone; fax):

Emergency contact (name; relationship; phone):

DOCTORS

SPECIALTY	NAME OF DOCTOR; ADDRESS	PHONE; FAX; E-MAIL
Primary care		
Surgeon		
Radiation oncologist		
Medical oncologist		
Other medical specialists you consult		

PRESCRIPTION MEDICATIONS

MEDICATION	DOSE	INSTRUCTIONS	PRESCRIBED BY

OVER-THE-COUNTER MEDICATIONS AND SUPPLEMENTS

MEDICATION (BRAND OR OTHER DESCRIPTION)	DOSE	WHAT YOU'RE USING IT FOR

Medical History

Date updated:

Name: Date of birth:

Address:

Phone: Fax: E-mail:

Hospital: Patient ID:

Insurance company: Insurance ID:

Allergies:

Pharmacy (name; phone; fax):

Emergency contact (name; relationship; phone):

Chronic lung disease	Other chronic illnesses
☐ asthma	☐ diabetes
☐ emphysema	☐ heart and circulatory conditions
☐ chronic bronchitis	☐ blood disorders
☐ other (explain)	☐ kidney disease
	☐ neurological problems
	☐ hepatitis
	☐ autoimmune disease
	☐ AIDS
	☐ other (explain)

Acute lung conditions Year	Previous surgery (cause, year)
☐ pneumonia ———	
☐ tuberculosis ———	
☐ collapsed lung ———	
☐ other (explain) ———	

Previous cancer (type, year)	Other medical events requiring hospitalization (cause, year)

Smoking status and history:	Family cancer history
Started at age _____	(relation, type of cancer, age at onset)
Ended at age _____	
Total pack-years _____	
☐ Exposure to passive smoke	

Other risk factors for lung cancer	Other illnesses or conditions that run in your family
☐ radon	
☐ asbestos	
☐ other (explain)	

Lung Cancer Treatment History

Date updated:

Name: | Date of birth:

Address:

Phone: | Fax: | E-mail:

Hospital: | Patient ID:

Insurance company: | Insurance ID:

Allergies:

Pharmacy (name; phone; fax):

Emergency contact (name; relationship; phone):

ORIGINAL DIAGNOSIS

Date: | Diagnosing physician:
Type, stage, and grade:

SUBSEQUENT DIAGNOSIS

Date: | Diagnosing physician:
Diagnosis:

TREATMENTS

Date: | Physician in charge:
Description of treatment:

Outcome:

Date: | Physician in charge:
Description of treatment:

Outcome:

Date: | Physician in charge:
Description of treatment:

Outcome:

Date: | Physician in charge:
Description of treatment:

Outcome:

CHAPTER 11

Surgery

If your doctors have recommended surgery as the initial treatment for your lung cancer, consider that very good news. Surgical removal of the tumor offers the best odds of a cure. But this kind of surgery isn't always possible, especially when lung cancer is advanced.

This chapter explains when and how lung cancer surgery is performed. We also provide practical information, from suggestions on selecting a surgeon to tips on speeding your recovery after the operation. At the moment, most people with lung cancer aren't eligible for potentially curative surgery. But we hope this will change soon, now that lung cancer can be found at a much earlier stage.

Is Surgery an Option?

Before you undergo surgery, your doctors will learn as much as they can about the extent and nature of your disease. They need to be sure—before they open your chest—that an operation is really appropriate. Sometimes the disease has advanced too far, or the tumor is in a position that makes an operation too dangerous. The doctors also will consider whether you're strong enough to tolerate such major surgery. The risk may be too great for someone who has significant heart or lung disease. If surgery isn't possible, the first treatment will be chemotherapy or radiation.

Small Cell Lung Cancer

Surgery is not ordinarily used to treat small cell lung cancer (SCLC), because people with SCLC usually have tumors throughout both lungs when they're diagnosed. But it may be an option if SCLC is found very early.

Non-Small Cell Lung Cancer

Surgery is the most common treatment for stage I or II non-small cell lung cancer (NSCLC). More advanced NSCLC usually is not treated surgically, but there are exceptions. Some patients with stage IIIA disease have cancers that can be removed completely. In other cases, stage IIIA or even IIIB patients can become candidates for surgery if they first have chemotherapy, radiation therapy, or both to shrink the tumor.

Surgery is more unusual for stage IV NSCLC, which has spread beyond the lungs. But it may be possible when both the primary tumor in the lung and the metastasized tumor are very small. Glenn was one of the lucky ones. By the time he was diagnosed, the disease had spread to his brain. In the hospital he glanced at his chart and read: "Lung cancer; three months to live." His first oncologist told him that nothing could be done beyond palliative care—measures to keep him comfortable. Glenn's wife insisted that they consult another doctor. Glenn speaks about what happened next:

> The new oncologist said, "Since you have one tumor in your lung and one brain metastasis, I might be able to do something curative." My heart soared. But he warned me: "If you have more metastases, there's nothing we can do." My wife got me in and out of all the tests, and there was just the one metastasis in my brain. They zapped that with radiation. A week and a half later, I had the operation. My entire right lung was removed. Later I had chemotherapy. That was four years ago, and I'm still in remission.

Selecting a Surgeon

All surgeons have specialized training that allows them to perform medical operations. Some are general surgeons; others specialize in specific proce-

dures, conditions, or parts of the body. As a rule, the more frequently surgeons perform a particular operation, the more skilled at that procedure they
are likely to be.

If you're facing surgery for lung cancer, we recommend that you select a
thoracic surgeon who specializes in lung surgery. Thoracic surgeons have
received extensive training in surgery of the chest, including the lungs and
heart, but some of them focus on lung surgery. If no specialist is available, try
to find a general surgeon who performs lung surgery often. See pages
148–149 for suggestions on locating doctors.

We suggest that you meet with more than one surgeon before you proceed. As we emphasized in Chapter 10, we also advise you to speak with at
least one radiation oncologist and at least one medical oncologist (specialist
in chemotherapy) to fully understand your treatment options. This is true
even if surgery seems clearly indicated, because chemotherapy and radiation
therapy may have key roles too.

See that copies of your medical records are forwarded to each doctor
before the appointment; deliver them yourself if time is short. It's helpful to
ask a friend or relative to accompany you on these visits so you can share
impressions.

Here are some issues to discuss with prospective surgeons:

- What are my alternatives to having this operation?

- Where will the surgery be performed? (A major cancer center or teaching hospital is best.)

- Who will actually operate? (If you're treated at a teaching hospital, make
  sure your operation will be performed by an experienced surgeon and
  not by a doctor-in-training.)

- How many times have you performed this particular surgery?

- What tests will I have beforehand? What will they involve?

- What will happen during the operation? How will my lymph nodes be
  checked?

- What complications might occur? Can I expect any problems because of
  my age or health status?

- What should I expect after surgery? Will I be in intensive care, and if so,
  for how long?

- How will my postsurgical pain be managed?

Specialists Versus Generalists

A team of researchers from the Medical University of South Carolina looked at records for all the lung cancer operations performed in the state from 1991 to 1995. Almost half were done by thoracic surgeons, the rest by general surgeons. Nearly all patients survived the surgery, but the death rate was significantly higher for those operated on by general surgeons. The differences were largest for those at highest risk because of their medical conditions or advanced age.

SOURCE: "Specialists Achieve Better Outcomes Than Generalists for Lung Cancer, Surgery," by G. A. Silvestri, J. Handy, D. Lackland, E. Corley, and C. E. Reed, in *Chest* 1998;114(3):675–80.

- How long am I likely to be in the hospital?
- What will the operation cost? How much will be covered by insurance?
- What can I do to speed my recovery after I leave the hospital?
- Should I have radiation or chemotherapy before or after surgery?

We believe that personal rapport is a significant issue when you're selecting a doctor with whom you will have an ongoing relationship, such as your primary care physician. However, you'll probably have only brief contact with your surgeon. So we suggest that you look for the most skilled and experienced surgeon available, even one whose bedside manner isn't ideal.

In addition to speaking with one or more surgeons, try to talk to other patients who have had the same procedure. Ask them to describe their experiences—what would they do the same way and what would they do differently?

Preliminary Tests

Before a lung cancer operation, you will undergo many tests—including pulmonary function tests—to make sure surgery is appropriate and safe for you. This greatly improves the odds of a successful outcome.

If You Use Supplements or Herbs

Be sure to tell your surgeon and anesthesiologist. Some supplements and herbs can be risky for a person who is having an operation, or they can alter the effectiveness of pain medication.

Tests to Evaluate the Cancer

Before your chest is opened, the surgeon must be certain that you really do have lung cancer and that the disease is *resectable* (can be surgically removed). If so, its exact location must be determined. Some patients still undergo major surgery after only a chest x-ray. That's not enough!

Here are some of the tests you may have before surgery. (See Chapter 8 for full descriptions.) Not every test is administered to every patient.

- Fine needle aspiration (needle biopsy), to obtain tissue samples from suspicious areas in the lungs

- Bronchoscopy of the central airways, to check for suspicious areas, determine their locations, and obtain tissue samples

- Imaging tests—such as x-ray, CT, MRI, and PET—to identify suspicious areas and check for metastases in the lymph nodes, brain, bones, liver, and adrenal glands

- Mediastinoscopy, usually performed under general anesthesia just prior to surgery, to examine the lymph nodes in the center of the chest

- Thoracoscopy, usually performed under general anesthesia just prior to surgery, to examine the lung periphery and lining of the chest

The best strategy for these preliminaries is to start with appropriate imaging tests and to follow up with the least invasive tests that are suitable for your particular situation. For example, if a PET scan finds distant metastases, you'll know immediately that surgery won't be the first treatment.

Despite preliminary tests, the surgeon still may find something unexpected when the chest is open and can be viewed directly. But careful preoperative assessment minimizes this possibility.

Overall Health Evaluation

You will be carefully checked to make sure that you can withstand the stress of an operation and that your lungs have enough reserve capacity to compensate for the loss of tissue. This can be an issue for people who suffer from other pulmonary conditions, such as emphysema or chronic bronchitis. If health problems would make an operation dangerous or would severely impair your breathing afterward, surgery is not appropriate. In that event, chemotherapy or radiation would be used instead.

Tests may include some or all of the following:

- Blood or urine tests to check for infections

- Cardiogram to assess the strength of your heart

- Blood tests to see how effectively your lungs and circulatory system distribute oxygen and disperse carbon dioxide

- Pulmonary function tests to determine if your lungs are strong enough.

Preparing for Surgery

You can take advantage of the brief time between diagnosis and surgery to improve your chances of a successful outcome. If you originally sought medical attention because you had signs of a respiratory infection, your doctor may prescribe a course of antibiotics. Other suggestions:

- **Quit smoking.** You'll increase the odds of a successful operation and reduce the chance that your cancer will recur. See Chapter 7 for information on smoking cessation.

- **Begin pulmonary physiotherapy.** The better the condition of your lungs, the more successful surgery is likely to be. Ask your doctor to refer you to a pulmonary therapist. Even brief pulmonary therapy can make a significant difference. Treatment might include aerobic exercise and breathing exercises to strengthen your respiratory muscles.

- **Try to get sufficient rest.** Relaxation exercises (see Chapter 15) may help if you have difficulty falling asleep during this stressful period.

- **Talk to a nutritionist about your diet.**

The Operation

Lung cancer surgery is performed in different ways, depending on the size and location of the tumor. But it's always a challenge for your body. During the operation you'll be under general anesthesia. Surgery usually lasts two to five hours. While you're anesthetized, but before your chest is opened, you may receive a bronchoscopy, mediastinoscopy, or thoracoscopy to check for the spread of cancer.

Types of Surgery

The surgeon will *resect* (surgically remove) the entire cancer along with surrounding healthy lung tissue, called a *tissue margin*. The margin is checked to make sure that the cancer has not spread beyond the resection.

The extent of the operation depends on how far the cancer has spread. Because the lungs are so much larger than needed to sustain life, a person can survive with just one lobe of a single lung. You may find it helpful to refer to

---

In Anticipation of Your Return Home after Surgery

- Stock the pantry and freezer; have ready-to-heat foods on hand, to minimize the need for shopping and cooking.

- Catch up on laundry, bills, cleaning, and other predictable chores to give yourself a break from household responsibilities as you recover.

- If your home has stairs, plan to have a bed on the first floor initially.

- Arrange for help. Ask your doctor if a home health aide is medically indicated. If so, insurance will pay for it.

- List tasks—cooking, cleaning, laundry, child care, shopping, and errands—that you can delegate to friends and family members who ask, "What can I do?"

What to Bring to the Hospital

Leave cash and valuables at home, but consider bringing the following for comfort:

- Earplugs and a sleeping mask so you can rest even if your roommate is watching TV or chatting with guests

- An inexpensive personal stereo with headphones

- Your favorite pillow in a distinctive pillowcase, marked with your name so it won't be confused with hospital linens

- Lip balm, since hospital air can be dry

- Pictures of your family

- Important telephone numbers and a phone card for long-distance calls

- Pad and pencil to take notes

- Bottled water if you're used to it

- Soft, loose-fitting clothing for the trip home

the illustrations of lung anatomy in Chapter 3 as you read the descriptions below.

The two most frequent surgeries are:

- **Pneumonectomy:** Resection of an entire lung. When cancer affects all the lobes on one side, the entire lung is removed.

- **Lobectomy:** Resection of a lobe. If the cancer is confined to a single lobe, only that lobe will be resected. If two out of the three right lobes are involved, both will be removed—that operation is called a **bi-lobectomy**. (The left lung usually has only two lobes; if cancer has spread to both, the entire lung is removed.)

Less common lung cancer operations include:

- *Sleeve resection:* Removal of a section of an airway and nearby tissue rather than a lobe. The procedure may be feasible if the tumor is in one of the main airways and has not spread deeply into a lobe. To picture it, imagine shortening the sleeve of a sweater by cutting away the worn-out elbow portion and sewing the remaining sections together. Though the operation is difficult to perform, a sleeve resection preserves more of the lung than a lobectomy does.

- *Extensive resections:* Removal of not only a lung or lobes but parts of the chest wall, ribs, the pleural membrane that surrounds the lungs, the diaphragm, and other affected areas. This is riskier than pneumonectomy or lobectomy, so patients must be carefully evaluated beforehand.

Entering the Chest

The general term for any operation that enters the chest is **thoracotomy**. Different kinds of incisions are used for lung cancer surgery, depending on the location of the tumor.

- **Side incision:** If the cancer is in the middle or lower portions of your lung, the surgeon probably will enter your chest between your ribs. The incision is likely to run under your arm, from your back to your front, but smaller incisions may be possible in some cases.

Why Not Remove Just the Tumor?

Lumpectomy is an accepted option for breast cancer, but not for lung cancer. Clinical research has compared lobectomy (removal of an entire lobe) to *limited resection*—operations that remove only the cancerous portion of a lobe and nearby tissue. Though more lung tissue is preserved with a limited operation, the average patient survival time is significantly shorter. Consequently, lobectomy is currently preferred. However, this could change with the use of CT scans, which can find much smaller tumors. More research will be needed to see if limited surgery is effective for these tiny tumors.

On the Horizon: Less Invasive Options

Watch for news of advances in lung cancer surgery as CT scans detect more early-stage tumors. Innovations under investigation, and already available at some centers, include:

- **Video-assisted thoracic surgery (VATS):** Rather than opening the chest to perform the operation, viewing and surgical instruments are inserted through small incisions between ribs. Because surgery is less invasive, recovery time is much shorter. But the surgeon may not be able to examine the chest cavity and lymph nodes as completely as can be done in standard surgery.

- **Photodynamic therapy (PDT):** Light is used instead of a knife to treat small tumors in the airways. A few days before the procedure, the patient is injected with a drug that makes cells much more sensitive to light. Normal as well as cancerous cells are affected, but the drug lingers longer in cancerous cells. A **laser** tool is inserted into the airway via a bronchoscope; the intense light of the laser targets the sensitized tumor. Afterward, the patient may experience temporary pain and breathlessness, but usually less than with surgery; recovery time is much shorter. Abnormal sensitivity to bright light continues for about a month. To prevent serious sunburn during that time, a person who has undergone PDT must be completely covered—including hands, face, and scalp—when going outdoors.

- **Front incision:** If the tumor is in the upper part of your lungs—or if the disease affects both sides of your chest—the incision probably will be made in front. The surgeon may make a vertical split in your **sternum** (or **breastbone**), the flat bone that runs from the bottom of your neck to the top of your abdomen. The cut also may run across your chest; or access may be gained by removing part or all of one or more ribs.

On the Horizon: Sentinel Node Sampling

An alternative to removing all the mediastinal lymph nodes could be *sentinel node* sampling, a procedure sometimes used for breast cancer surgery. The sentinel node is the first lymph node into which a tumor drains. Injecting the tumor with dye and tracking its movement into the lymphatic system identifies this node. Preliminary studies in lung cancer patients suggest that if the sentinel node shows no sign of cancer, the other lymph nodes are cancer-free and need not be removed. However, more research is needed to compare survival with sentinel node sampling and complete lymph node dissection.

Checking for Metastases

No matter how carefully you're evaluated beforehand, there's no substitute for a direct examination. Before anything is removed, your lungs, the chest cavity, and the lymph nodes of the mediastinum will be checked.

The surgeon will *palpate* (examine by touching) the lymph nodes; those that are larger and harder than normal are more likely to be cancerous. But even an experienced surgeon might miss a small tumor. Because of this possibility, most thoracic surgeons perform a *complete lymph node dissection*. In other words, they remove all the lymph nodes in the mediastinum. Studies show that this practice improves the odds of survival. Nevertheless, surgeons who are not thoracic specialists sometimes remove only some of the lymph nodes when they treat lung cancer patients. Discuss this issue ahead of time with your surgeon, especially if you don't have a thoracic surgeon.

Occasionally, despite appropriate preliminary tests, the surgeon finds much more extensive cancer than expected. Sometimes the disease is too widespread to permit surgery. In that case, the incision will be closed without removing any portion of the lung, and plans will be made for radiation or chemotherapy instead.

The Role of Pathology

Before surgery proceeds, samples will be taken from the tumor, nearby lung tissue, and lymph nodes. Portions of these samples will be quick-frozen in liquid nitrogen, sliced into very thin sections (called *frozen sections*), and stained to highlight any cancerous cells. The sections are rushed to the pathology laboratory while the anesthetized patient waits on the operating table. The pathologist—a doctor who specializes in tissue examination and laboratory tests—checks the samples and reports immediately to the surgeon. Once the surgeon knows what's cancerous and what's healthy, the operation can continue.

A preliminary pathology report will be available immediately after the surgery. When you wake up from anesthesia, the surgeon will be able to tell you what type of lung cancer you have and if there are signs that it has spread to your lymph nodes. You'll also be told if the margins—the border of normal tissue around the tumor—appear to be cancer-free. Further analysis will be performed on the remaining tissue samples over the next day or two, and a full pathology report will be sent to your doctor. (See page 116.)

Recovery

After the operation, you'll be taken to the hospital's intensive care unit (ICU), where you'll be watched closely in the initial hours of your recovery. When you wake up from surgery, you'll find yourself attached to many devices:

- Monitors to check your lung and heart function

- Oxygen delivery system to assist your lungs

- Drainage tubes in your chest to remove excess air and fluid

- A catheter for urine

- An intravenous line (IV) to provide nutrition and medication

- A catheter to allow blood tests without need for additional needle pricks

If all goes well, you'll probably be moved from the ICU to an ordinary hospital room within twenty-four hours. You'll be urged to sit up and begin to walk (with assistance) as soon as possible. Over the next few days, you'll be weaned off oxygen; the drainage tubes, IV, and catheters will be removed.

Most people remain in the hospital for four to seven days after lung cancer surgery, depending on the specific operation performed and their overall health as well as on the practices at their hospital and the rules of their insurance plan or HMO. However, hospital stays may be longer if an infection develops or if you're weakened by other medical problems. By the time you go home, you should be able to breathe and walk on your own. Here are suggestions for getting your recovery off to a good start:

Arrange for Effective Pain Management

Discuss postoperative pain with your surgeon before the operation. Ask if the hospital has a team of pain management specialists—many teaching hospitals do. If so, arrange to speak with someone from this team.

Effective pain management is not just for your comfort; it also is a matter of health. Studies have found that proper pain relief actually speeds recovery and shortens hospital stays. You'll be able to breathe better and to work harder on rehabilitation if pain is controlled. On the other hand, too much pain medication can interfere with pulmonary function. One particularly effective approach is *patient-controlled analgesia* (PCA), in which pain medication is delivered in tiny doses when you press on a button. (See box on page 296 for more on PCA.)

Comfort Tips for Incision Pain

Postsurgical pain around the incision usually becomes less severe after a week or two, but some people are troubled by lingering pain or loss of sensation. Our advice:

- Tell your doctor if you're having pain near your incision. You might have an infection or you might need a change in pain medication.

- Wear soft, loose clothing.

- For women: If the incision is at your bra line and you are reluctant to go braless, consult a bra specialist who works with breast cancer patients after mastectomy.

- Consider treatment with acupuncture, which may be helpful. Acupuncture is increasingly available in hospitals, which means you can start immediately after surgery.

Comfort Tip for Coughing

Your lungs will accumulate excess fluid after surgery, which creates a threat of pneumonia. While you're in the hospital, the pulmonary therapist will encourage you to cough and clear out the fluid. But when you cough, you may feel that your incision is about to pop. The solution: Use a pillow to provide gentle support as you cough. For a front incision, hold the pillow against your chest and fold your arms across it. For a side incision, tuck the pillow under your arm and press it against your side. If the incision was made in your back, lean against the pillow.

Begin Exercising as Soon as You Can

While you're in the hospital, discuss exercise with your doctor. For someone who's just had an operation for lung cancer, "exercise" means getting out of bed, sitting in a chair, and walking to the bathroom. The sooner you start moving again after surgery, the sooner you'll feel like yourself. But this won't be easy at first.

Ask your doctor for a referral to a pulmonary rehabilitation therapist. The therapist will encourage you to turn from side to side, breathe deeply, cough, and walk as soon as you're able. These activities help your remaining lung tissue return to normal.

Avoid Infection

During the weeks after surgery, as your body recovers from the traumas of anesthesia and a major operation, you are more vulnerable to infection than usual. Be scrupulous about personal hygiene, and stay away from anyone who has a cold or other contagious illness.

Getting Back into Shape

Full recuperation typically takes at least four to six weeks. However, it's not unusual for lung cancer patients to find that they don't regain their former

Breathing Muscle Trainer

An inexpensive hand-held device called an *inspiratory muscle trainer* can improve your breathing. Think of it as bodybuilding for the muscles involved in respiration.

The trainer consists of a mouthpiece attached to a tube. You block your nose with a clip and exhale into the mouthpiece. A valve controls the challenge of pushing air through the tube. As your muscles get stronger, the setting can be increased.

Talk to your doctor or a respiration therapist about using an inspiratory muscle trainer. The trainers are sold by prescription, but they're inexpensive (about $10 to $25) and may be covered by insurance. One source is the Allergy Supply Company, 11994 Star Court, Herndon, VA 20171; 800-323-6744 or 703-391-2011; *http://www.allergysupply.com.*

energy for six months to a year after surgery. Try not to be discouraged or impatient. You'll probably see significant improvements in a matter of weeks, even if you're not yet back to normal.

Becoming Active Again

Rehabilitation exercises can be very helpful (we suggest a few below). Even more important is your overall level of activity throughout the day. You may feel tempted to stay in bed, but try not to become an invalid. Think of your bed as a place for sleep; minimize the time you spend there when you're awake. As your strength returns, graduate from sitting to walking. Go outdoors once or twice a day if you feel up to it and if weather permits.

―――――

After surgery to remove my right lung, I was in the hospital for twelve days. I went home and was in bed for two weeks. Then I got a call from a client saying, "We have a job." I hauled my butt out of that bed and hobbled down to the job interview. I got the job and went to work. It was good for me.
  —Glenn

Stretching and Strengthening Exercises

During periods of inactivity, your body loses flexibility and muscle tone. Two exercises for your arms, wall walks and arm lifts, will help you recover. These exercises are appropriate for most people in the first days and weeks following lung cancer surgery. Once you've mastered them, you'll be able to move on to more vigorous activities that can further strengthen your lungs.

Before you start, check with your doctor.

Rehabilitation Exercises

A full program for rehabilitation after lung cancer surgery usually includes three kinds of exercises:

- **Breathing exercises** that expand the lungs and work the muscles involved in respiration. See pages 28–29, 178, and 255.

- **Stretching and strengthening exercises** that improve flexibility and strength. See pages 179–182.

- **Aerobic activity** that works the heart and lungs. See suggestions for a walking program on page 74.

You can start belly breathing as soon as you wake up from surgery, while you're still in intensive care. Ask your doctor when you can begin other exercise. Usually it's safe to start gentle stretching and strengthening exercises while you're still in the hospital. You'll also be encouraged to walk as soon as possible.

After you return home and as your recovery continues, you can begin aerobic exercise—workouts that speed your heart and make you breathe faster. At the beginning you might not be able to manage more than a slow, brief walk. Your capacity will increase if you persist. Push yourself a little, but get sufficient rest and don't overdo. You'll know that you've struck the right balance if you make good progress toward recovery without setbacks from exhaustion.

First some general instructions, then the exercises:

- Begin with the wall walks. The wall supports your arms as you extend your range of motion.

- When the wall walks become significantly easier, change to arm lifts, which involve similar moves but without wall support.

- When you're ready to increase the challenge further, use light weights for the arm lifts.

- Work at proper intensity. As you do the exercises, your arm muscles should become fatigued. If your muscles don't feel tired after you do the exercises, increase the effort a little as described below. With normal muscle fatigue, any mild discomfort disappears within minutes after you stop. If that doesn't happen, or if the exercise is actually painful, you may be pushing ahead too quickly.

- Use belly breathing (see page 28–29) as you do the moves.

Wall Walks

Do the front wall walk. Pause for a minute or two to rest, and then do the side wall walk.

FRONT WALL WALK   Stand or sit facing a wall. Place your left hand on the wall at the height of your waist.

- Walk the index and middle finger of your left hand up the wall, while inhaling through your nose. Reach as far over your head as possible. With each repetition try to move higher up the wall.

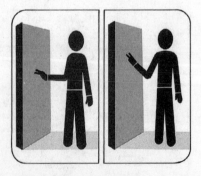

- Walk your left hand back down the wall to the starting position while slowly exhaling through your mouth.

- Change hands and repeat. Work up to a total of 10 repetitions on each side. Try to go a little higher each time you do the exercise, until you can extend your arm all the way up.

SIDE WALL WALK   Stand or sit with your left side toward the wall. Place your left hand on the wall at the height of your waist.

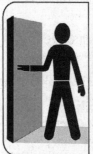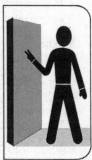

- Walk the index and middle finger of your left hand up the wall, while inhaling through your nose. Try to reach as far over your head as possible.

- Walk your left hand back down the wall to the starting position while slowly exhaling through your mouth.

- Repeat 10 times (or as many times as you're able). Turn so that your right side is facing the wall and do the same moves with your right hand. Work up to a total of 10 repetitions on each side.

Arm Lifts

These exercises are more challenging because your arms support themselves. The moves will further improve the strength and flexibility of your chest and arms.

SIDE ARM LIFT   Sit in a chair with your arms down at your sides.

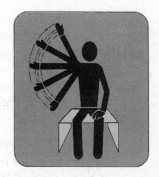

- Slowly raise your right arm up and to the side, while inhaling through your nose. Reach as far to the side and as high as possible.

- Slowly lower your arm back to the starting position while exhaling through your mouth.

- Work up to a total of 10 repetitions with each arm.

- When one-arm lifts become easy, do the side lift with both arms.

- Next, add a slow body-twisting move at the top to increase flexibility in your spine: When your arms are shoulder-high, bring one arm forward and the other back. Reverse the two arms to twist to the other side.

FRONT ARM LIFT   Sit in a chair with your arms down at your sides.

- Slowly raise both arms forward and above your head, while inhaling through your nose. Reach as far over your head as possible.

- Slowly lower your arms back to the starting position while slowly exhaling through your mouth.

- Work up to a total of 10 repetitions.

TWISTING ARM LIFT   Sit in a sturdy chair that has no arms. Place your left hand on your right knee.

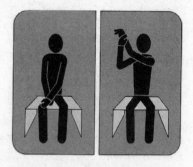

- While inhaling through your nose, slowly lift your left hand and arm up and as far to the right as possible. If necessary, use your right arm for support.

- Exhale through your mouth while slowly lowering your arm back to the original position, with your left hand on your right knee.

- Switch sides so that your right hand is on your left knee and repeat, moving your right hand and arm up while stretching to the left. Repeat, working up to a total of 10 lifts on each side.

When the arm lifts are no longer difficult, you can increase the challenge by adding light hand weights. Begin with a 1-pound weight (you can use a 1-pound can, provided you can easily grasp it in your hand). When lifting that becomes easy, use a 2- or 3-pound weight; gradually increase further as you become stronger. At this point it's safer to use hand weights than cans because they're easier to grip securely. Inexpensive hand weights are available at many discount stores and sporting good stores.

Medical Follow-up after Lung Cancer Surgery

Everyone who has lung cancer surgery hopes for a cure—and indeed, surgery offers the best chance for that. Unfortunately, there's still a possibility that some cancer cells were missed. This is true even if your surgeon told you, "I got it all." Also, anyone who's had lung cancer once is at risk for a recurrence. So it's essential that you arrange for appropriate follow-up monitoring. That means regular checkups, including CT scans. We'll give details in Chapter 16.

If you haven't already had your case reviewed by a medical oncologist and a radiation oncologist, we urge you to do that now. Though surgeons don't always suggest this, it's very important to consult a medical oncologist about the advisability of chemotherapy after surgery. In 2003, a large international study showed for the first time that chemotherapy improved survival after surgery for early-stage lung cancer.

If the tissue margins were not cancer-free, many surgeons will recommend radiation. Be sure to talk to both a medical oncologist and a radiation oncologist to find out what they suggest. If possible, have your case discussed by a tumor board—a meeting in which several specialists review the case and give their opinion. Ask if you can be present during this discussion.

The recovery process will continue after you come home from the hospital. Be patient with yourself. It takes at least a few weeks—and often many months—to regain your strength and energy.

CHAPTER 12

Chemotherapy

Cancer cells were found in fluid removed from my lungs. A week later I had diagnostic surgery to find out how advanced it was. Afterward, I was in the recovery room and the surgeon went to the waiting room. My husband, his boss, two close family friends, the assistant pastor from our church, my parents, and my sister were there. The surgeon told them, "The cancer has moved beyond her lung into the lining of her chest. There's really nothing we can do." Everyone was devastated.

My sister is a nurse. She asked, "Should we even consider chemotherapy?" The surgeon was very pessimistic. He said, "You'll have to decide if you want her to go through that."
—Donna P.

Donna—only 36 at the time of her diagnosis, with a husband and young daughter—was determined to fight. For seven years, she was victorious. During that time she underwent nine chemotherapy regimens plus radiation therapy. Some of her chemotherapy treatments were tough, with nausea, hair loss, and a metallic taste in her mouth that was so powerfully unpleasant it woke her up at night. But in the weeks and months between treatments, Donna traveled with her husband, worked, participated in her community—and thoroughly enjoyed her life. Most important of all, she saw her daughter grow from age 10 to age 17.

Chemotherapy is still tragically underused against lung cancer. Many well-meaning doctors discourage people with advanced disease from pursuing chemotherapy. Patients often dread the side effects more than the cancer. A 1999 survey commissioned by the Oncology Nursing Society asked new cancer patients to identify their greatest concern. Thirty-two percent said that they were worried about whether they'd survive. But more—40 percent—said that their biggest concern was the side effects of chemotherapy.

If you feel the same way, you should know that chemotherapy is now much more tolerable than it used to be. Special medications and improved timing of doses can counter nausea and other side effects. Numerous studies show that chemotherapy not only increases longevity, but also improves the quality of life. This chapter explains how chemotherapy is used and how it works. We also provide many practical suggestions for making treatment as safe and comfortable as possible.

Terms and Timing

- *Induction chemotherapy* refers to chemotherapy given as the first treatment. Sometimes only chemotherapy will be used; sometimes radiation or surgery will follow.

- *Neoadjuvant chemotherapy* is given *before* surgery or radiation. This form of induction chemotherapy is intended to shrink the tumor so that it becomes small enough to treat with surgery or radiation.

- *Concurrent* or *combination chemotherapy* refers to chemotherapy used at the same time as radiation therapy. The drugs make the tumor more sensitive to radiation.

- *Adjuvant chemotherapy* is given *after* surgery or radiation. Its purpose is to kill any remaining cancer cells.

- *Consolidation chemotherapy* is a second round of chemotherapy administered after an initial round to kill any cancer cells that may have survived the first treatment.

Do You Need Chemotherapy?

We recommend that everyone diagnosed with lung cancer consult a medical oncologist before deciding on a treatment plan. Such a consultation is important even if you've already had surgery or radiation. Chemotherapy isn't prescribed for everyone with lung cancer, but it's used for some patients at all stages and with all types of the disease.

Small Cell Lung Cancer (SCLC)

Treatment of small cell lung cancer nearly always includes chemotherapy. With limited-stage SCLC, the goal might be to cure the cancer. If the disease has spread, chemotherapy is used to slow its progress and to relieve symptoms.

Non-Small Cell Lung Cancer (NSCLC), Stages I and II

The standard care for stages I and II NSCLC is surgery alone. But we now know that even the very small tumors found by CT are sometimes metastatic. This means that when small stage I or II tumors are removed, undetectable cancer cells may remain behind in the lungs, lymph nodes, or other sites. Even successful surgery—and even a negative PET scan or other imaging test—doesn't guarantee that all the cancer has been removed. Some oncologists believe that postsurgical chemotherapy can help prevent recurrences; others disagree. Clinical trials are underway to settle the question.

Non-Small Cell Lung Cancer (NSCLC), Stages III and IV

Chemotherapy is the most frequently used treatment for NSCLC at stages III and IV. It may be given alone or in combination with surgery, radiation, or both.

Stage IIIA

If the cancer has spread within the chest, but is still on the same side as the affected lung, the best hope for a cure or long-term survival is a combination of treatments. Sometimes it begins with chemotherapy to shrink the tumor before surgery or radiation. Chemotherapy also may be used after surgery or radiation to kill any remaining cancer cells.

Stage IIIB

At this stage, both sides of the chest are involved but the cancer has not spread to other parts of the body. A combination of chemotherapy and radiation offers the best hope for long-term survival. After this initial treatment, surgery may be possible. Chemotherapy may be used after the operation also, as a safeguard against invisible cancer cells.

Stage IV

When cancer has spread beyond the chest, the disease usually is not curable. Chemotherapy—alone or with radiation—is used to relieve symptoms and extend survival time. We want to emphasize that we're not talking about gaining a few miserable weeks in the hospital. ALCASE is in touch with many patients who have lived with stage IV disease—and lived well—for five years and longer. They think of lung cancer as a chronic disease. Chemotherapy halts or slows the growth of their tumors. If the tumors begin to advance again, another round of chemotherapy is prescribed. Sometimes the treatments have unpleasant side effects. But between these brief periods, these long-term survivors enjoy extra years of fulfilling life.

How Chemotherapy Works

Chemotherapy treats cancer by killing malignant cells or preventing them from dividing. Since cancer cells divide more frequently than normal cells, they're more vulnerable to chemotherapy drugs. These drugs work by different mechanisms. You can think of them as vandals, saboteurs, and decoys:

- "Vandals" damage the DNA of cancer cells.

- "Saboteurs" interfere with mechanisms necessary for cell division.

- "Decoys" mimic essential enzymes or nutrients, depriving cancerous cells of substances they need to survive and divide.

Chemotherapy *protocols* (treatment plans) for lung cancer often include two or three types of drugs. That's because multiple attack routes can be more effective against the disease.

Drugs Used for Lung Cancer Treatment

The most common chemotherapy protocols use platinum-based drugs—carboplatin (Paraplatin) and cisplatin (Platinol)—or newer agents such as docetaxel (Taxotere), gemcitabine (Gemzar), irinotecan (Camptosar), paclitaxel (Taxol), topotecan (Hycamptin), and vinorelbine tartrate (Navelbine). Drugs are often used in combination to kill more cancer cells.

The newest drug treatments are called biologic agents, because they mimic the body's own chemicals. One example is gefitinib (Iressa), a growth factor inhibitor (see box on page 197), which was approved by the Food and Drug Administration in 2003.

The specific regimen you receive will depend upon what's currently recommended for your type and stage of lung cancer, as well as on your doctor's preferences. Recommendations change frequently, as researchers test one drug treatment protocol against another.

Why Side Effects Occur

Unlike surgery and radiation therapy, which target a single site, chemotherapy affects the entire body. The good news is that it can destroy cancer almost anywhere it has spread (the brain and bones are exceptions), even if growths are too tiny to be visible. But there's a downside, which is that healthy cells may be damaged too. Especially vulnerable are:

- Cells that normally divide rapidly, such as bone marrow cells, hair follicles, and cells in the lining of the mouth and intestinal tract

- Sensitive cells, such as those in the nervous system

- Any cells that happen to be dividing during treatment

In most cases the normal cells can recover, so the problems are temporary. Also, medications can counter most side effects, at least partly, making chemotherapy tolerable.

Timing and Dose

Chemotherapy usually is given in cycles with rest periods in between. The goal is to kill as many cancer cells as possible, while allowing normal cells time to recover. The specific therapies you're given—the drugs used, the schedule, and doses—depend on the stage and type of your disease and your other medical conditions. These therapies are developed and refined on the basis of clinical trials with many patients. That's why it's important to stick with the schedule even if it conflicts with other important events in your life, and with the dose even if it causes some side effects. Treatment may be modified, however, as your doctors observe your response.

Preparing for Chemotherapy

We've already made suggestions about selecting a doctor and listed questions to ask. (See Chapter 10.) At your first meeting with your medical oncologist, you'll also address the following concerns about chemotherapy:

- What drugs are available to treat my form of cancer? Which are considered best?

Supportive Care

Measures that help counter the side effects of treatment are called *supportive care.* The better your supportive care, the safer and more effective your treatment will be. Unfortunately, doctors don't always offer the best available treatments. They may be unfamiliar with them, or the drugs may be expensive.

Don't suffer needlessly. Insist on supportive care, even if you pride yourself on being a stoical, undemanding patient. These measures are as much a part of high-quality chemotherapy as are cancer-killing drugs.

- What drug or drugs will I be taking? (If they're not the same as the ones considered best, find out why they're being used.)

- Where will I receive treatment?

- How many treatment sessions will I have, and how long will they last?

- How will the drugs be administered?

- How will treatment benefits and side effects be monitored?

- What are the common side effects of this treatment?

- When am I most likely to experience these effects?

- What supportive care can you offer to minimize side effects?

- Are there any problems that I should report immediately?

- What are my options if this regimen doesn't work?

If possible, visit the treatment facility—the place where you will actually receive chemotherapy—before your first session. It may be part of your doctor's office, a separate clinic, or a department at a nearby hospital. This will give you an opportunity to meet the oncology nurses and to talk with patients about their experiences. Find out the best way to schedule your chemotherapy sessions. Savvy patients book appointments well in advance to obtain the most convenient time slots or private rooms.

See Your Dentist Before Treatment

Chemotherapy can make the lining of your mouth more vulnerable to irritation, sores, and infection. Have your teeth cleaned before you begin treatment. Explain that you will be starting chemotherapy for cancer. Ask the dentist to check your teeth, gums, and dentures (if you wear them) and to address any problems. If you need dental work during chemotherapy, ask your oncologist if any special precautions are necessary—and be sure to tell the dentist about your cancer treatment.

It was scary to see how the nurses handled the chemicals. I said to them, "You're wearing gloves and vests to protect yourself from this chemical that you're putting into my body?"
—*Glenn*

How Chemotherapy Is Administered

You'll probably have chemotherapy on an outpatient basis. However, a short hospital stay might be necessary at the beginning to monitor your reactions to the drugs and make any necessary adjustments.

Most chemotherapy for lung cancer is administered intravenously—that is, through a vein. (Administration of medication or other fluids through a vein is called an **infusion**.) Some new drugs can be taken orally, in pill or liquid form. But usually this is not possible: the drugs might irritate the digestive tract or the digestive system might interfere with their action.

The first day of chemotherapy I cried the whole time. Of course, I knew I had lung cancer. But in the back of my mind I had been thinking, "This must be a dream. There has to be some mistake." Now I was hooked up to the IV and I knew it was for real. The nurse gave me a box of tissues and said, "Don't worry about crying. A lot of people cry on the first day."
—*Donna P.*

Intravenous Chemotherapy

One way to administer intravenous chemotherapy is to insert the needle into a vein in your hand or forearm each time you have a treatment. But this may be risky for certain toxic drugs, which could burn your skin. Also, some drugs are more effective when they're delivered to larger blood vessels. And of course, repeated needle pricks can be uncomfortable, especially if your veins are small or hard to reach.

Port and Catheter

Port
A metal or plastic disk is implanted under your skin. Attached to the inside is a thin, flexible tube that is threaded into a large vein in your chest. This device— the disk and the tube—is a port.

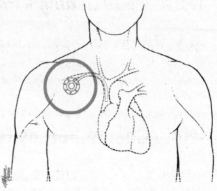

Catheter
A catheter is similar to the tube part of a port. One end is inserted into a vein, but the other end hangs outside your body instead of connecting with a disk just under your skin.

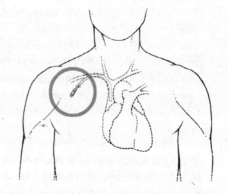

An alternative is to use a port or a catheter, either of which is implanted semipermanently in your chest during a minor outpatient surgical procedure and can be removed after treatment ends. Chemotherapy is administered through the device instead of through a needle in a vein. Most patients find this easier. Also, the drug can't leak out and hurt the skin. Your oncologist and oncology nurse can help you decide what's best. For additional information, see the articles about ports at *http://www.cancerlynx.com/nurseport.html* (click on the additional links at the bottom of the page to read patient messages).

Tip: If You're Getting a Port or Catheter

Though the device must be near the blood vessel, you may be able to select the specific location with comfort and appearance in mind. For example, you might prefer a spot that can't be seen when you wear an open-neck shirt. Or if you're a woman, you might ask to have the port or catheter installed above or below your bra line to avoid chafing.

My veins are very deep and very small, and they were difficult to find for chemotherapy. I was having a lot of anxiety about the needles. My doctor suggested a port in my chest. With the port, the nurses could get a sure hit every time. But they had to go through the skin in my chest to get to the port, which was painful. After my first round of chemotherapy, I had the port removed.

The second time I had chemotherapy, I got a catheter. The tube hung out of my body and I tucked it into my bra. At night I was afraid I'd roll over on the tube and pull it out when I was sleeping. Cleaning it every day was a hassle. Also, I couldn't go swimming with it. But the injection was more comfortable—they just put it in the tube.

For the third round of chemotherapy, I went back to the port. I would put EMLA anesthetic cream on the area one or two hours before chemotherapy; that helped a lot with the needles. I've had the port for four years. Eventually my skin became tough enough so that I no longer need the cream. There's nothing for me to clean or maintain. Once a month I go in for blood tests. They take blood through the port and they flush the port to clean it.

—Donna P.

Pills and Liquids

Sometimes chemotherapy or supportive care drugs are administered orally. If you're going to take pills or liquids, discuss the medication with your oncologist or oncology nurse. Some questions to ask:

- Is it best to take the medication with a meal, after a meal, or on an empty stomach?

- Should I avoid any foods, nutritional supplements, or other medications that might interfere with its action?

- If nausea or drowsiness are expected in my case, can I take the drug at night rather than in the morning?

Even if you normally swallow pills easily, it may be difficult if your mouth becomes dry or sensitive during treatment, or if the medication has an unpleasant taste. Here are some suggestions:

- If the medication tastes bad, numb your taste buds first by sucking on ice chips or sherbet.

- Pack unpleasant-tasting pills into empty medicine capsules, which are available at most drugstores and health food stores; you won't be able to taste them.

- If your mouth is dry or sensitive, lubricate it with a few sips of water before taking pills.

- Ask your doctor or pharmacist if the medication can be given in a form that's easier to swallow—perhaps smaller tablets or a liquid instead of a tablet.

- Find out if hard-to-swallow pills can be crushed. If so, you can crush them into applesauce or jelly to make them easier to get down. (Note: Some pills lose efficacy if they're crushed, so it's important to ask your doctor or pharmacist.)

Dealing with Side Effects

All of the chemotherapy drugs used to treat lung cancer cause side effects in some people. Your doctor will explain what reactions are likely, based on the particular drugs you'll receive and the experience of other patients. Of course, your response might be quite different.

During chemotherapy, tell your doctor and oncology nurse about any symptoms that emerge. One reason is that much can be done to make

> ## The Importance of Fluid Intake During Chemotherapy
>
> **C**hemotherapy is toxic—that's how it kills cancer cells. These poisons will be flushed out through your kidneys and bladder. If you don't drink enough liquids, your kidneys and bladder will be exposed to higher concentrations of toxic chemicals. That's why you'll be given beverages during treatment and told to keep fluid intake high. Drinking can be difficult if you're nauseated—yet another reason to keep nausea under control.

chemotherapy safer and less unpleasant. But you can't assume that every new problem is related to chemotherapy. The change could have another cause—including tumor growth—so it needs to be checked out.

Below are some of the common side effects of chemotherapy. You may not experience any of these difficulties. Few people suffer from all of them.

―――

A lot of people go into chemotherapy thinking they're going to be ill. Your perception fuels reactions. For me, it was very pleasant. My wife came with me every time. She brought our children to the first appointments so doctors could see I had a young family that needed me.
—Glenn

―――

Hair Loss

When newly diagnosed lung cancer patients ask about chemotherapy, the first question is usually: Will I lose my hair? For many people, hair loss (the medical term is *alopecia*) is one of the most traumatic side effects of chemotherapy. It's a visible reminder of the disease to ourselves and to others. Your doctor can tell you if hair loss is a common side effect of your chemotherapy drugs.

On the Horizon

Chemotherapy is improving all the time. Below are a few new approaches that currently are under investigation. Some are already available via clinical trials (see Chapter 14).

- **Tests that predict which chemotherapy drugs will be most effective:** Some tumors resist chemotherapy; some individuals are particularly sensitive to toxic effects. Researchers are working on genetic tests that could help predict these reactions so doctors can better customize treatment to the individual.

- **New ways to administer chemotherapy:** Existing treatments may be significantly more effective or have fewer side effects if they're administered differently. One experimental approach is inhaled chemotherapy for lung cancer, which delivers drugs directly to the lungs. Treatments take just ten minutes. Another new approach is daily chemotherapy. Currently, chemotherapy is given in the highest doses patients can tolerate, using supportive care and breaks in

Hair cells, like cancer cells, divide rapidly. So they're also vulnerable to chemotherapy. When hair loss occurs, it usually begins one to four weeks after treatment starts. Sometimes only the hair on your head is affected, but you might also lose hair elsewhere on your body.

Fortunately, hair loss can be camouflaged—and it's temporary. Typically, hair begins to grow back when chemotherapy ends. Formerly curly hair may now be straight (or vice versa); the color may be different. It may take up to a year for your hair to return to its normal length, color, and texture. Or the change may be permanent.

———

I cried the day my hair started to fall out, even though I knew that was going to happen. I called my husband at work, and he came right home. My husband is bald. He said, "If anyone can relate to what you're going through, I can."

treatment to manage side effects. Under investigation is a new tactic that reduces side effects: giving smaller doses every day.

- **Less-toxic drugs:** Researchers are investigating drugs that fight cancer without the toxicity of traditional chemotherapy. One very promising new approach involves *anti-angiogenesis drugs*, which destroy the blood vessels that develop to nourish cancerous tumors. If this new blood supply is successfully blocked, the tumor starves to death. Dozens of anti-angiogenesis drugs are being tested alone or in combination with chemotherapy. Another exciting development is the use of *growth factor inhibitors* in cancer treatment. Growth factors are substances in our body that encourage cells to grow and replicate. Sometimes they contribute to the spread of cancer. Certain drugs that inhibit particular growth factors have been highly effective in clinical trials.

- **New medications to counter side effects:** When side effects are reduced, patients can tolerate higher and more effective doses of chemotherapy.

The hair loss was tough, but I dealt with it. I wore a wig to work and church. At home I liked to wear a comfortable cap a friend gave me that said, "Bad hair day." My hair had been straight and blondish, with light brown highlights. When it grew back it was darker, thicker, and had waves.
—Donna P.

———

Here are some suggestions for dealing with hair loss:

- Before hair loss starts, be gentle with your hair and scalp. Avoid hair dryers, curling irons, and electric curlers. Ask your doctor if it's safe to have your hair dyed or waved.

- When you sleep, wear a soft night cap to protect your hair. If shedding begins, the cap will contain it.

Paying for a Wig

- Contact your insurance company or HMO; many insurers cover the cost of a wig if hair loss is caused by illness or medical treatment.

- Contact a local cancer organization or support group. Some have free "wig banks."

- If you expect to pay for your wig, ask your doctor for a prescription indicating that the wig is *a hair prosthesis required because of hair loss caused by cancer treatment.* Save a copy of your prescription and receipt for income tax time; the IRS considers this a legitimate medical deduction.

- Consider cutting your hair short. Some people prefer to shave their scalp when hair loss begins. They want to take control of the process and get it over with quickly.

- If you decide to buy a wig, buy it before chemotherapy so you can match your hair color. Or try a new color you've always liked. Ask your local cancer organization for a referral to a wig salon that specializes in chemotherapy patients. Remember that a wig—like your own hair—needs to be washed and cared for to look its best.

- Experiment with other head coverings, such as turbans and scarves.

- If you decide to go bald, wear sunscreen to protect your scalp when you're outdoors. In cool weather, wear a hat, since considerable body heat is lost from a bare head.

The loss of other hair—eyebrows, eyelashes, and hair in the nostrils—is not conspicuous, but it creates problems too: your eyebrows and eyelashes help protect your eyes from dirt in the air; nostril hair traps dust and microorganisms before they reach the lungs. Some suggestions:

- Wear protective eye coverings, such as glasses or goggles.

- If your nose drips more than usual because you don't have nostril hairs, keep tissues handy. A light coating of petroleum jelly (one popular brand is Vaseline) may help prevent both infection and dripping.

- Learn to use makeup to conceal loss of eyebrows and eyelashes. Women can contact the American Cancer Society's Look Good, Feel Better program (800-395-LOOK; *http://www.lookgoodfeelbetter.org*). Or call your local ACS office.

Nausea and Vomiting

Many people believe that chemotherapy inevitably causes nausea and vomiting (also called *emesis*). This is one of the most dreaded side effects of cancer treatment. In fact, not all chemotherapy drugs produce nausea. Even drugs known to have this effect on some patients don't affect everyone the same way. What's more, new medications can block or at least reduce the problem.

What Causes Vomiting and Nausea

You might assume, based on unpleasant experience, that vomiting and nausea are problems of the stomach. But they're actually triggered by special centers of the brain. Neurotransmitters—chemicals that act on nerve or muscle cells—are released by cells in the gastrointestinal tract that are susceptible to chemotherapy drugs. These neurotransmitters stimulate the nausea and vomiting centers. Some drugs tend to produce immediate nausea; with others, nausea sets in the day after chemotherapy. Individual sensitivities are a factor too.

Preventing the Problem

Discuss nausea and vomiting with your oncologist before treatment starts. At stake is your health as well as the quality of your life. Uncontrolled nausea can have serious medical consequences, including weight loss, dehydration, malnutrition, and weakness. Severe vomiting can tear the digestive tract or open surgical wounds. Patients debilitated and demoralized by nausea and vomiting may give up treatment that might have cured them.

Preventing the problem is much easier than getting it under control once it starts. That's why antinausea medication should be given before you begin chemotherapy and continued long enough to counter delayed nausea.

Drugs Used to Prevent Nausea and Vomiting

Patients who are starting chemotherapy sometimes are offered metoclopramide (Reglan) or prochlorperazine (Compazine). These are older, relatively inexpensive drugs that help some people. But three newer drugs—dolasetron (Anzemet), granisetron (Kytril), and ondansetron (Zofran)—are more likely to be effective. If you know you're vulnerable to nausea (one clue is that you get motion sickness) or if your chemotherapy protocol usually causes severe nausea, ask your doctor to prescribe one of the newer medications, even though it's more expensive.

If these don't work, other drugs may be tried, including dronabinol (Marinol), droperidol (Inapsine), or lorazepam (Ativan). Dronabinol is the active ingredient in marijuana. In some parts of the United States, it's legal to use marijuana for medicinal purposes. Research suggests that it's not as effective for most people as the newer antinausea drugs. However, marijuana sometimes relieves nausea in individuals who are not helped by other measures.

These measures should not be taken "as needed": if nausea is allowed to develop, the drugs will be much less effective. Indeed, some people develop anticipatory nausea: they become nauseated or vomit *before* chemotherapy. This is usually a conditioned response to previous treatment in which antinausea measures were inadequate.

You may need to try several medications or a combination of drugs before you get relief. Don't give up! Let your oncologist and oncology nurse know if you're experiencing nausea, especially if you're vomiting so much that you can't keep liquids down. The cause is probably the chemotherapy. But sometimes cancer patients develop nausea for tumor-related reasons, so it could be a significant symptom.

Practical Tips

You may experience queasiness even with antinausea medication. Here are simple measures that may reduce the problem:

- Adjust your diet. Avoid fried or fatty foods. Eat and drink slowly. It's often better to consume smaller amounts more frequently.

- Keep your house filled with fresh air. If cooking odors provoke nausea, minimize them by cooking ahead, buying prepared foods, or accepting a friend's offer to provide dinner. Since food has a stronger aroma when it's hot, select items that can be eaten cold or at room temperature.

- Counter nausea by sucking hard candies or sipping clear beverages, including apple juice or noncaffeinated sodas that have lost their fizz.

Effects on Eating and Digestion

Good nutrition helps maintain your strength during chemotherapy, but eating well becomes a challenge. Your appetite may disappear; food may not taste right. Treatment also may produce constipation or diarrhea. That's because the drugs affect cells in the intestinal tract; in addition, chemotherapy may kill some of the beneficial bacteria that aid digestion. Emotions affect eating and digestion too. Though it's difficult not to be anxious if you're being treated for lung cancer, try to minimize unnecessary stress. Relaxation techniques may be helpful (see Chapter 15).

See page 73 for a brief summary of dietary recommendations from the American Cancer Society and the National Cancer Institute. Also see their excellent free booklets, which offer information and recipes:

- *Nutrition for the Person with Cancer: A Guide for Patients and Families*, by the American Cancer Society. Order by calling 800-ACS-2345.

- *Eating Hints for Cancer Patients Before, During, and After Treatment*, a publication of the National Cancer Institute. Available online (*http://www.cancer.gov/cancerinfo/eatinghints*) or in print (call 800-4-CANCER).

Loss of Appetite

Talk to your doctor or oncology nurse if you find you can't eat. The cause is probably chemotherapy, but there could be another reason, such as depression or fatigue, both of which can be addressed. If the problem persists and you're losing too much weight, food supplements like Ensure or Sustacal can provide basic nutrients and calories. Or your doctor might suggest a medicine that stimulates appetite and builds lean body weight.

Constipation

Constipation is a common problem during chemotherapy. Sometimes it's a side effect of the drugs or other medications; sometimes it's the result of chemotherapy-related changes in eating or a consequence of inactivity.

If you become constipated, call your doctor or oncology nurse. They may suggest dietary modifications or prescribe stool softeners and laxatives. Don't take medicine—not even over-the-counter remedies—without checking first. Also ask before adding high-fiber foods to your diet; this may not be appropriate if your white blood cell or platelet counts are low.

Diarrhea

Call your doctor if you develop diarrhea that persists for more than twelve hours or that is associated with cramps or bleeding. Check before using medication. Deal with the problem promptly, not only because it's unpleasant but also because it can lead to dehydration and loss of nutrients. In the meantime, prevent infection by being scrupulous about bathroom hygiene.

Pampering a Delicate Appetite

- Avoid the effort and odors of cooking. Ask other people to fix your meals, or use prepared food.

- Eat when you're hungry rather than being guided by customary meal times and menus. For instance, if you're able to eat well in the morning, enjoy a dinner-size breakfast.

- If you can manage small quantities of food, eat frequently throughout the day rather than having three large meals.

- Add calorie-boosting ingredients to your usual fare. For instance, add nuts to stir-fries, salads, and casseroles; top vegetables with cheese.

- Drink beverages between meals rather than along with food, since fluids make you feel fuller.

- Try stimulating your appetite by taking a walk before you eat.

The evening after my second chemotherapy treatment I went to bed feeling fine. In the middle of the night I awakened. There was something warm between my legs. I had defecated. I'm alone and it's all over me. I get myself to the bathroom and jump into the shower with my nightgown on. I'm sniveling. I can't believe this is happening to me. I get myself all cleaned up. Then I'm nauseated. I look up in the mirror over the toilet. I see this ancient crone with no hair, vomiting in the toilet. I cried. Who is this person in the mirror? It isn't me. This is all a terrible dream. I washed the sheet in the sink. Then I had to shower again and make the bed up.

Now I'm prepared every time I have chemotherapy. I put one of those blue plastic sheets on the bed, just in case. But it never happened again.

—Anita

Effects on Bone Marrow (Myelosuppression)

Chemotherapy can damage the **bone marrow**, the tissue inside bones where blood cells and other components of blood are produced. The result is **myelosuppression:** reduced bone marrow activity that results in fewer white blood cells, red blood cells, and platelets. ("Myelo" comes from the Greek word for marrow.) After chemotherapy, blood components usually return to normal or near normal. But with each successive treatment, bone marrow may rebound less effectively.

Many people haven't heard of myelosuppression before they start chemotherapy, though they're aware of possible hair loss and nausea. But myelosuppression can be far more serious. At its worst, it can be life-threatening. Indeed, myelosuppression is the side effect most likely to be **dose limiting**—that is, it can limit the dose or frequency of your chemotherapy. Myelosuppression also can drain your energy, produce mental confusion, and make you vulnerable to painful infections.

Doctors counter myelosuppression with three basic approaches:

- By delaying or reducing the dose of chemotherapy. Unfortunately, studies show that this reduces the effectiveness of treatment.

- With blood transfusions. This is an effective measure, but only temporarily. Moreover, it exposes patients to infection and other risks from blood transfusions.

- With *growth factor treatments*, medications that boost blood cell production. This is the best way to prevent and counter myelosuppression. Though these drugs are costly, they usually allow chemotherapy to proceed on schedule.

During chemotherapy your blood will be checked regularly to see if it contains normal quantities of white and red blood cells and platelets. This test is called a *blood count*. Ask to see the results rather than waiting for symptoms; your oncology nurse can explain what the numbers mean. If myelosuppression becomes a problem, ask if growth factor treatments could help.

Leukopenia (Insufficient White Blood Cells)

Our white blood cells normally defend the body against a variety of dangers, from precancerous cells to infectious microorganisms. Different kinds of white blood cells tackle different threats. The type that specializes in fighting germs is the **neutrophil**. This is the kind of white blood cell most likely to be affected by chemotherapy. If we don't have enough of these warriors—a condition called **neutropenia**—we become more vulnerable to infections. The best way to prevent and control neutropenia is with a growth factor called G-CSF (Neupogen), which stimulates production of neutrophils.

Because your immune system may be weaker than usual during chemotherapy, take special care to prevent infections:

- Avoid crowds; stay away from people with contagious illnesses.

- Wash your hands before eating, after using the bathroom, and after blowing your nose.

- Observe food safety cautions with particular care. Don't eat undercooked meat, fish, or poultry; wash fruits and vegetables; refrigerate perishable items.

- Don't share towels, drinking glasses, or silverware with others. Use the hottest water cycle in your dishwasher to kill germs.

During cancer treatment, take signs of infection very seriously. Call your oncologist immediately if you develop any of the following seemingly minor problems—symptoms you might normally treat on your own:

- Fever over 99 degrees Fahrenheit

- White patches or painful areas in your mouth

- Pain, redness, or swelling near the injection site or elsewhere on your skin

Your doctor won't think you're overreacting. In fact, don't be surprised if you're told to come to the office or emergency room immediately.

Mouth Sores and Other Oral Problems

Organisms that live in the mouth—bacteria, viruses, yeasts, and fungi—are normally controlled by white blood cells. But they may proliferate if you have leukopenia. The result can be oral infections like thrush, ulcers, or canker sores. These painful conditions can develop very quickly. Tell your oncologist immediately if you notice sores or other problems in your mouth. Your doctor may prescribe medication or suggest home remedies. Prevention tips:

- See your dentist for a cleaning and checkup before you start treatment.

- Use a soft, clean toothbrush and a toothpaste that contains sodium bicarbonate to reduce the acid in your mouth. Avoid anti-plaque toothpaste and mouthwash, which may be irritating. Floss gently.

- Avoid acidic, spicy, or very hot foods, which may irritate sensitive tissues.

- Drink plenty of water. Chew gum to stimulate saliva flow. If necessary, lubricate your mouth with glycerin swabs, synthetic saliva sprays, or a water-based lubricant such as K-Y jelly.

Anemia (Insufficient Red Blood Cells)

Red blood cells carry oxygen through the body. Having too few red blood cells—anemia—is like having a reduced air supply. Symptoms include shortness of breath, lethargy and fatigue, headache, dizziness, and pallor. People who suffer from chemotherapy-related anemia may feel so tired that they can't work and can't think clearly. Note that fatigue can have other causes, including stress or tumor growth. Tell your doctor if you're abnormally tired so that appropriate treatment can be prescribed.

Chemotherapy-related anemia can be treated with red blood cell transfusions, which bring immediate relief. But this is just a temporary fix and it involves the risk of infection. Better, though much more expensive, is a growth factor called erythropoietin (Procrit, Epogen). Erythropoietin is a hormone produced by the kidneys that stimulates bone marrow to make more red blood cells. (You may have heard about this drug if you follow sports news, because some athletes secretly use it to boost their performance.)

A less common cause of anemia among people undergoing chemotherapy is iron deficiency. This could occur if your diet becomes inadequate as the result of nausea or loss of appetite. If iron deficiency is diagnosed, it can be treated with iron supplements or dietary improvements.

Thrombocytopenia (Insufficient Platelets)

Platelets are the component of blood that enables it to clot. If your platelet count is low you're vulnerable to bruising, nosebleeds, and uncontrolled bleeding. Thrombocytopenia can be treated with platelet transfusions. As with red blood cell transfusions, the improvements are rapid but temporary. The superior approach is to use interleukin-11, a blood cell growth factor that helps the bone marrow create more platelets.

If you know your platelet count is low, take care to avoid injuries that could cause bleeding:

- Avoid contact sports and physical activities that increase your risk of falling.

- Use an electric shaver, not a razor. Don't clip your nails—maintain them with a file instead.

- Postpone nonessential dental work, including cleaning. Use a soft toothbrush (or a child's toothbrush) that doesn't make your gums bleed.

Neurological Effects

Chemotherapy often affects nerve cells. This can produce side effects throughout the body, from mental confusion to tingling in the toes. Here are the most common neurological problems:

Peripheral Neuropathy

When chemotherapy damages the nerves of your arms and legs, the result can be peripheral neuropathy. The problem usually starts with tingling (a pins-and-needles sensation) in the fingers and toes. It may extend to the feet and hands, and progress to pain or a complete loss of sensation.

Tell your doctor if you develop tingling in your hands or feet. If the problem becomes troubling, ask about amifostine (Ethyol). Ongoing research suggests that the drug may be able to relieve or prevent these symptoms.

Peripheral neuropathy usually disappears gradually when chemotherapy ends. In the meantime, physical and occupational therapy are helpful for managing symptoms and coping with disabilities. A few tips:

- To simplify dressing, use clothing or shoes that close with snaps, zippers, or Velcro instead of buttons or laces.

- Check out the gadgets designed to help people with arthritis perform everyday tasks like getting dressed, cooking, and writing. These are available at many pharmacies or medical supply stores. One good mail-order source is Dynamic Living (888-940-0605; *http://www.dynamic-living.com*).

- For more information about peripheral neuropathy, read *Numb Toes and Aching Soles: Coping with Peripheral Neuropathy*, by John A. Senneff (Medpress, 1999).

▬▬

No one warns you about the neuropathy. Your hands become almost useless. You can't button yourself properly, and it's hard to hook a necklace around your neck. It's almost impossible to open a bottle of Snapple. I was assured that this would slowly go away and some of it did. But there's a residual neuropathy.
    —Anita

▬▬

Peripheral neuropathy makes people accident-prone and clumsy. If you develop the problem, examine your hands and feet daily to make sure you haven't injured yourself and take these precautions:

- **In the kitchen:** Anything that can become dangerously hot—stoves, cooking equipment, food, or water—presents risks to someone who has impaired sensation in the hands. Wear protective oven mitts to handle anything that might be hot.

- **In the bathroom:** Adjust the thermostat of your water heater to prevent burns, or use a thermometer to check water temperature. Install bathmats and hand rails to minimize the risk of falls.

- **Around the house and in the office:** Since the loss of feeling in the feet affects balance, eliminate hazards such as loose rugs and clutter. Improve lighting if possible, and add hand rails to stairs that don't already have them.

- **In the car:** Be aware that your driving ability may be impaired if you lose sensation in your feet. Remove your shoes when you drive so you can feel the pedals.

- **Outdoors:** Avoid exposure to cold, since you could suffer frostbite without knowing it.

Mental Confusion

Almost everyone who receives chemotherapy talks about the "chemo-fuzzies"—small problems of mental clarity, such as faulty memory and difficulty concentrating. The problem isn't in the brain itself, because most chemotherapy doesn't reach the brain in large amounts (that's why radiation or surgery must be used for metastases to the brain). Rather, there's damage to nerves elsewhere in the body, so the signals that reach the brain aren't clear enough. Fortunately, these effects usually diminish after chemotherapy ends, though it may take as long as a year for full recovery.

If you experience mental changes during treatment, bring them to the attention of your medical team. The cause is probably chemotherapy, but the same symptoms can result from anemia or from the spread of the disease.

I fumble for words and for the names of people I know. Sometimes it's like playing charades to coax words out of me. My kids say, "Mom, you're just having a senior moment." No—it's different.
—Anita

Hearing Problems

Chemotherapy can damage nerves that affect hearing. The result can be ringing in the ears, hearing impairment, or increased sensitivity to noise. Usually the problem improves gradually after treatment ends, but sometimes the damage is permanent. Report the problem to your doctor and ask for treatment suggestions. Amifostine (Ethyol) may be helpful; some patients have told ALCASE that acupuncture is beneficial.

Fatigue

Most people experience fatigue during chemotherapy. As we explained earlier in this chapter, fatigue can be caused by anemia. Another reason is that your body is repairing the tissue damage caused by chemotherapy, a process that demands considerable energy. The problem may be exacerbated by nausea and resulting poor nutrition, as well as by emotional stress. And the cause could be lung disease or a tumor.

Tell your doctor and oncology nurse if you experience unusual fatigue. For more information about cancer-related fatigue, see Chapter 17.

Other Side Effects

Your doctor will look for side effects—including changes in cardiac or liver function—during your checkups. Here are other problems you may notice. Mention them to your oncologist or oncology nurse, and ask for suggestions about dealing with them.

- Changes in taste and smell; a metallic taste in your mouth

- Changes in skin, including sun sensitivity, and in fingernails or toenails

- Sexual changes, including loss of libido, erectile dysfunction in men, and increased vaginal dryness in women

For More Information

Here are resources for additional information about chemotherapy:

- *Chemotherapy and You: A Guide to Self-Help During Cancer Treatment* is a superb free booklet from the National Cancer Institute that offers comprehensive information about treatment and possible side effects, as well as helpful advice about coping. For a free copy, call 800-4-CANCER; the booklet is available online at *http://www.cancer.gov/cancerinfo/chemotherapy-and-you.*

- Lung Cancer Online (*http://www.lungcanceronline.org/effects/chemoeffects.html*) has comprehensive links to information about chemotherapy, including links to fact sheets on specific drugs that provide details about side effects.

If you have lung cancer and your doctors suggest chemotherapy, we hope you won't hesitate to accept it out of fears based on outdated information. Today's chemotherapy is less arduous—and more effective—than the chemotherapy of twenty years ago. And over the next twenty years, we expect even more improvements.

CHAPTER 13

Radiation Therapy

Radiation therapy, sometimes called radiotherapy, is the treatment of cancer and other diseases with x-rays and other penetrating rays. These rays can kill cancer cells or damage them enough to prevent them from dividing and proliferating. Unlike chemotherapy, which affects the entire body, radiation therapy can be aimed directly at cancerous tissue. And while it can target tumors inside the body, it doesn't involve an invasive surgical procedure.

More than half of people diagnosed with lung cancer receive radiation therapy, most often when the disease is at an advanced stage. Sometimes radiation is the only treatment, but usually it is part of a plan that also includes surgery, chemotherapy, or both. This chapter will explain how radiation therapy works and how its special capabilities contribute to lung cancer treatment. We'll offer suggestions for maximizing the benefits and minimizing side effects.

How Radiation Therapy Works

Radiation is all around us. Our bodies are constantly bombarded by different kinds of radiation from natural and manufactured sources, including radio waves, microwaves, x-rays, gamma rays, cosmic rays, and light. Of these, light is most familiar. You probably know that sunlight contains different kinds of radiation, including not only visible light but also infrared radiation (the rays that make sunlight feel warm) and ultraviolet radiation (the component that causes sunburn). You also know that the effects of light vary with its intensity: strong sunlight can burn your skin, while a dim light merely illuminates. However, even the brightest light can't reach below the skin, and its radiation can be blocked by thin materials like fabric or paper.

The invisible rays used for cancer treatment—x-rays, gamma rays, and electrons—behave similarly to light in some respects. But these rays can penetrate deep inside our bodies; it takes a thick barrier of lead to stop them. They're beamed into the body at low intensity to create diagnostic images, such as chest x-rays. At the much higher intensity used for radiation therapy, the same rays can damage or destroy cells.

Radiation treatment damages cells along the path of the rays. Cancer cells hit by radiation usually die or become unable to divide. Normal cells may be affected too, but they can recover, just as healthy skin can recover from a sunburn. Cancer cells are less able to repair themselves.

How Radiation Therapy Is Used

Radiation has a role in treating lung cancer at all stages. Sometimes it's used alone; sometimes it is teamed with other measures. We recommend that you consult a radiation oncologist before deciding on a treatment plan. Even if you've already had surgery or chemotherapy, it's not too late for this important input.

Small Cell Lung Cancer (SCLC)

Small cell lung cancer generally involves multiple tumors, so the main treatment is chemotherapy. If the disease is found at the limited stage—while it's still confined to one lung and the mediastinum (area between the lungs)—a combination of chemotherapy and radiation therapy has been shown to give the best chance for a cure. Radiation may be used to sensitize tumors so they're more vulnerable to chemotherapy drugs. Or radiation may be given as **consolidation therapy** after chemotherapy, to kill or disable any remaining cancer cells.

When SCLC has reached the extensive stage (has moved beyond the chest), chemotherapy alone is the preferred initial treatment. If chemotherapy fails to halt its spread, radiation may be used to treat selected cancerous areas that are causing pain, breathlessness, or other distressing symptoms. Radiation is particularly valuable for treating SCLC that has spread to the brain, bones, or spine. Radiation of the brain (*cranial irradiation*) is used not only to treat metastases but also to prevent them. The preventive procedure, called **prophylactic cranial irradiation (PCI)**, has been controversial because benefits are limited and there is significant concern about side effects. However, recent studies convincingly show that PCI significantly increases the odds of disease-free survival for small cell lung cancer patients whose disease has been successfully treated in the chest. Side effects—the most significant of which is diminished mental capacity—can be reduced by waiting to give radiation until after chemotherapy is completed.

Non-Small Cell Lung Cancer (NSCLC)

Currently, radiation is used mostly for advanced NSCLC. But it may become increasingly important in treating early NSCLC as more very small tumors are found with CT scans.

Stages I and II

Most patients with early-stage lung cancer are treated with surgery, since that offers the best chance for a cure. But radiation may be used instead when surgery isn't possible—for example, if the patient is unable to withstand a major operation or when a tumor is too close to the heart, major blood vessels, or major airways.

Radiation may be given before surgery (*neoadjuvant therapy*) to shrink the tumor. The role of radiation treatment after surgery (*adjuvant therapy*) is controversial for people with stage I or II disease. Proponents point out that invisible cancer cells may remain after surgery; radiation could kill them and prevent the disease from coming back. But some studies suggest that radiation treatment doesn't improve survival. Your own radiation oncologist will make a recommendation based on the characteristics of your disease.

Stage III

Radiation therapy is used frequently at stage III, often with other treatments. When NSCLC has moved beyond the lung but is still on one side of the chest (stage IIIA), treatment may begin with surgery; afterward, radiation, chemotherapy, or both are given to kill any remaining cancer cells. If surgery isn't possible because of the size or position of a stage IIIA cancer—

or if the disease is at stage IIIB (cancer is on both sides, but still confined to the chest)—treatment will start with chemotherapy, radiation, or a combination. Sometimes (more often with stage IIIA than IIIB) the aim is to shrink the tumor to operable size. In a smaller number of cases, the hope is that radiation or chemotherapy, together or alone, can cure the cancer or at least halt its growth.

Stage IV

When lung cancer spreads outside the chest, curative treatment usually isn't possible. But there are rare exceptions. For example, a person with a small lung tumor might have surgery to remove that, while radiation therapy tackles a tiny lesion in the brain. Chemotherapy may be used as well, to kill any invisible metastatic tumor cells.

More commonly, the treatment goals for stage IV patients are to contain the disease and improve quality of life. Radiation therapy, alone or with chemotherapy, can play an important role. It's often used to shrink inoperable tumors that cause pain, breathlessness, or other symptoms. If the tumor is localized, these problems can be addressed rapidly with radiation, sparing the patient the side effects of chemotherapy or the stress of surgery.

When lung cancer has metastasized to the brain, radiation is usually the treatment of choice: surgery would be much more invasive and chemotherapy is thwarted by the **blood-brain barrier**, special blood vessels that prevent most chemicals from entering the brain. Similarly, radiation is valuable for bone metastases. Surgical treatment—removing the tumor and surrounding bone—would dangerously weaken the skeleton and cause considerable pain; chemotherapy is usually too slow because bone cells divide more slowly than other tissues in the body (that's why a broken bone takes so much longer to heal than a cut in the skin).

━━━

I was diagnosed with lung cancer seven years ago and have been treated off and on with chemotherapy. Last spring I developed shortness of breath when I was going up the stairs in my house; I'd also have to slow down to catch my breath when I was walking. My doctors hadn't wanted to give me radiation therapy before, because I'd lose lung capacity. But now my right lung was ninety percent filled with tumors. Also, tumors at the bottom of the lung were encroaching on my liver.

Starting in the summer of 2000, I had about forty radiation treatments. They treated my right lung, the mediastinum (area between the lungs), and the mass near my liver. Within a week, I had less shortness of breath.
        —Donna P.

▬▬

Selecting a Radiation Oncologist

Chapter 10 has general suggestions about selecting a doctor. When you look for a radiation oncologist, the treatment facility is a significant consideration too. Medical oncologists generally have access to the latest chemotherapy

---

A Guide to the Radiation Professionals

R adiation therapy is always a team effort. These are the professionals who work together to provide your treatment:

- **Radiation oncologist:** A physician with specialized training in treating cancer with radiation therapy. The radiation oncologist is the team leader.

- **Radiation physicist:** A professional with training and expertise in the equipment used to deliver radiation therapy.

- **Dosimetrist:** A technician who calculates the time each treatment should last to deliver the radiation dose prescribed by the radiation oncologist.

- **Radiation technologist:** A technician who positions you and administers treatment.

- **Radiation nurse:** A nurse with training in radiation therapy who coordinates treatment and answers questions.

Do You Take Nutritional Supplements?

Tell your doctor about all of the medications you take, including over-the-counter drugs, herbal remedies, and nutritional supplements. Some doctors believe that high doses of antioxidant vitamins—such as vitamins A, C, or E—may make radiation therapy less effective.

drugs and protocols, regardless of where they practice. However, the situation is different for radiation oncologists, who rely on very expensive equipment. The technology available to treat you can vary considerably from one facility to another. Convenience is an issue too, since radiation therapy usually involves daily treatments over a period of weeks. Even if you can't leave home for that long and must select a radiation oncologist in your own community, consider getting a second opinion from a radiation specialist at a major cancer center. One form of radiation therapy, *radiosurgery*, which we'll discuss below, usually involves no more than a few treatment sessions, so travel might be practical.

In addition to the general questions you'd ask any doctor (see pages 149–51), here are specific questions for your radiation oncologist:

- What kind of treatment do you recommend?

- What other options do I have?

- What will treatment accomplish for me? Is the aim to cure my cancer? Or is the hope to slow its growth or relieve my symptoms?

- Can anything be done to make this treatment more effective? For example, would I get better results if I had chemotherapy as well?

- What is the schedule of treatments? How long will each session last? Can the timing be adjusted to my work schedule or to other personal plans?

- What side effects can I expect, and when are they likely to occur?

- What can be done to relieve or prevent these side effects?

External Radiation Therapy

Radiation therapy for lung cancer usually is given externally: high-energy rays are directed into your body to reach the tumor. The radiation may be generated by a **linear accelerator**, a machine powered by electricity; or a natural source of radiation—such as **cobalt-60**, a radioactive version of cobalt that emits gamma rays—may be used. The beam may target a single tumor and a **tissue margin** (the border of apparently healthy tissue around the tumor). Or radiation could be aimed at an area that might harbor invisible cancer cells, such as the section of a lung from which a tumor was removed. The skin through which the beam passes is called the **radiation port** or **radiation portal**. The rest of your body is shielded from the rays.

In planning your treatment, the radiation oncologist will consider the characteristics of your cancer. Tumors—because of their size, their doubling time (the number of days between cell divisions), their blood supply, or other factors—are not equally sensitive to radiation. Another concern is the vulnerability of nearby normal tissues. The wider the area that receives radiation and the higher the dose, the greater the chances of killing all the cancer, but the more likely that normal cells will be damaged too. All these issues must be balanced to determine the type of external radiation therapy you will receive, the dose to be used, and the schedule for treatment.

One recent improvement is **three-dimensional conformal radiation therapy**. Using advanced x-ray technology and computer image construction, the location, shape, and dimensions of a lung tumor are mapped. Radiation beams are directed from multiple angles to converge on the tumor. The cancer receives a large dose of radiation from all the beams, while surrounding normal tissue receives much less. This is especially valuable when tumors lie close to the heart, the esophagus, or other structures that are particularly sensitive to the rays.

The Treatment Schedule

Your medical team will determine the total amount of radiation needed to treat your tumors. Since normal cells will be affected too, the full amount won't be given in one session (unless you're having a single radiosurgery treatment). Instead, the total dose is divided into **fractions**, which are administered in daily treatments over four to eight weeks. The length of time over which radiation is given is referred to as **protraction**.

Stereotactic Radiosurgery

Stereotactic radiosurgery—a high-dose version of three-dimensional conformal radiotherapy—may be offered to patients whose cancer is confined to a single small area. Like ordinary surgery, stereotactic radiosurgery targets tumors exactly. But there's no anesthesia and no cutting. Since the radiation is very precisely focused, side effects usually are lower than with conventional radiotherapy. At the same time, doses can be higher, which allows treatment to be completed in just a few sessions instead of daily sessions over a period of weeks. Stereotactic radiosurgery is performed with systems based on a linear accelerator (for example, the X-Knife, CyberKnife, or Peacock system) or a cobalt-60 machine (Gamma Knife).

When stereotactic radiosurgery is feasible, it's often the best way to treat brain metastases from lung cancer; sometimes whole-brain radiation is used too. However, radiosurgery is not always appropriate and not all radiation oncologists have the necessary training or equipment. If you have a small brain tumor and stereotactic radiosurgery isn't

The radiation dose is usually the same for each session. But there are variants. For example, radiation therapy may be *hyperfractionated:* the dose is divided into very small fractions, with treatments given as frequently as every four to six hours. Sometimes the total dose remains the same, but each individual dose is smaller in the hope of reducing side effects. Hyperfractionation is also used to permit a higher total dose or a more rapid treatment schedule, with the aim of improving efficacy. One obvious drawback of hyperfractionation is that it's inconvenient for the patient and sometimes for the staff as well. Clinical studies are comparing different treatment plans to determine which are most effective for which kinds of lung cancer.

What to Expect During Radiation Therapy

On the first day, before radiation therapy actually begins, you'll go through a very important process called *simulation.* The radiation oncologist will map the exact area to be treated and plan how to best direct the radiation offered, try to get additional opinions from doctors experienced with this technique.

Radiosurgery is currently used most often for small brain tumors. However, new techniques and equipment increasingly permit its use for lung tumors as well—a very exciting development that will mean much less debilitating treatment for the patients with very early lung cancers found by CT.

———

Since I had a single lesion in my brain, I was referred for Gamma Knife surgery. They fasten a helmet to your head. You lie on a table and they slide you into a chamber that covers your neck and head. It's scary, but it's only for about twenty minutes and there's a panic button. The radiation doesn't hurt, but there's some pain from the helmet. They give you Tylenol and that does the trick.

I have an MRI every three months. For a year, my lesion continued to get smaller. Then it started to get bigger. They zapped it and it started shrinking again. Now the lesion is staying steady.
—Ben

to treat your tumor, while avoiding sensitive tissue. Think of it as a dress rehearsal for treatment, with a beam of laser light standing in for radiation.

During simulation you'll lie on an examining table with form-fitting foam cushions or other devices to keep you in a fixed position. If you're having radiation treatment for your brain, your head may be immobilized by a special helmet or mask. The tumor will be located by CT, MRI, or ultrasound. Tiny dots will be tattooed or marked on your body to help technicians position the beam exactly the same way each time you're treated.

Simulation can take an hour or more. If you're having radiosurgery, in which radiation usually is given in a single dose, treatment will follow simulation. Otherwise, you'll probably begin radiation treatments the next day. Each appointment will last about fifteen minutes to half an hour. But nearly all of that time is spent preparing and checking. The radiation therapist will use the marks on your skin to position you. You'll be held in place with cushions or other devices, as you were for simulation. However you won't need a lead apron as you do for a dental x-ray, because the beam used for radiation

---

Tips for Comfort and Effectiveness

Your radiation oncology team will warn you not to use powder, lotion, or deodorant. Even a seemingly innocuous product like baby powder might interfere with the radiation beam. Here are additional suggestions:

- Wear comfortable, loose-fitting clothing. Your skin may become more sensitive as radiation therapy continues, so select soft fabrics.

- Since you may have to wait, bring a friend or something to divert you—a book, magazine, or personal stereo.

- Between treatments, take care not to wash off the marks placed on your skin to help position the beam.

---

therapy is much more focused. The actual treatment takes just a few minutes. The technician will leave the room when radiation is administered, but can hear and see you at all times. You won't feel anything, though you will hear noise from the machine.

Over the weeks of treatment, your radiation oncologist will monitor your progress and address any side effects; if necessary, the schedule or dose can be adjusted. Unless you're experiencing severe fatigue or have been told not to drive (a precaution suggested for some people who have brain metastases), you probably can drive yourself to and from radiation sessions. Some people wonder if radiation therapy makes them radioactive. No, it does not.

Internal Radiation Therapy: Brachytherapy

Radiation therapy also may be delivered internally, a form of treatment called *brachytherapy*. Instead of using a large machine as the radiation source, a small amount of radioactive material is placed inside the body— near or in a tumor, or in an area from which a tumor has been removed.

Brachytherapy dates back to the 1950s, when Dr. Ulrich Henschke (Claudia Henschke's father) experimented with it.

Brachytherapy is used much less frequently than external radiation to treat lung cancer. It can be valuable in late-stage disease for quickly relieving symptoms of an airway tumor, such as severe breathlessness or coughing. However, the procedure has a high rate of complications, including bleeding (which can be life-threatening) and damage to the airway. Your radiation oncologist can tell you if it's recommended in your specific situation.

When brachytherapy is used for a tumor in an airway, the procedure is usually performed under sedation and local anesthesia. A long, thin, flexible catheter is threaded into the airway under the visual guidance of a broncho-scope. Radioactive material in the form of pellets or a thin wire is placed next to the cancerous tumor via the catheter. If you have high-dose brachytherapy, this material remains next to the cancerous tissue for ten to fifteen minutes, and then it is removed along with the catheter; treatment usually involves two to four sessions about a week apart. With low-dose brachytherapy, the radioactive substance and catheter remain in place for a few days. During this time, you will be hospitalized.

Special precautions are followed during brachytherapy to protect others from the radioactive material that is treating your cancer. The medical staff may work behind a shield or wear special gloves. If you're having low-dose brachytherapy, you'll be hospitalized in a private room and visiting will be limited. Once the radioactive wire or pellets are removed from your body, these precautions are no longer necessary.

Radiation Side Effects

Chemotherapy affects your entire body. But most side effects of radiation therapy are limited to the area that has received radiation. Some side effects appear during treatment; these are usually temporary. However, other prob-lems—called late side effects—may develop months or even years after radi-ation treatment is finished. These effects may be permanent.

In planning treatment, consideration will be given to your prognosis. When the treatment goal is improved quality of life in advanced disease, the focus is on relieving current symptoms even at the risk of long-term side effects.

Fatigue

The most common side effect of radiation therapy is fatigue. Most people experience some degree of fatigue after two weeks of radiation treatments. The feeling may gradually increase as treatment continues. Fatigue usually begins to wear off within a week after therapy is finished, though it may take weeks or months to disappear entirely.

On the Horizon

Radiation therapy is constantly improving, thanks to innovations in both equipment and technique. Here are some of the new approaches:

- **Body radiosurgery:** Stereotactic radiosurgery, already widely used for brain metastases, hasn't been used as much for lung tumors because the lung moves with every breath and normal tissue could be damaged. But new techniques are getting around that problem. One method is to immobilize the patient with a body frame. Yet another possibility under investigation is to implant a radioactive seed in the periphery of the tumor so its movement can be tracked by computer and instant adjustments made in the beam.

- **Sensitizing and protecting drugs:** Experimental drugs may make radiation more effective while minimizing side effects. *Radiation sensitizers* selectively make cancer cells more sensitive to the damaging effects of radiation. *Radiation protectors* shield normal cells from damage, permitting higher doses of radiation to be used against tumors.

- **Radioactive antibodies:** Some cancer cells trigger the immune system to produce antibodies. These antibodies can be produced in the laboratory in great quantity and then attached to radioactive substances. When the special antibodies are injected into the body, they selectively seek out tumors—and the radiation destroys them. This treatment approach, still at the experimental stage, is called *radioimmunotherapy*.

The main reason for fatigue is that your body is building tissues to repair the damage done by radiation, a process that demands energy. This effect is magnified when the tissue involved is lung tissue. Of course, fatigue also may be related to other aspects of the disease, to conditions like emphysema or chronic bronchitis, or to the stress of having cancer and the need to make daily trips for radiation therapy.

———

The radiation treatment itself is a piece of cake. It takes ten minutes at most. One side effect was fatigue. It hit me over the head from the first dose, and it was monumental. Other fatigue is treatable: when you're tired, you take a nap or get a night's sleep. Those things do not work with radiation fatigue. You're just as tired when you get up from taking that rest. You're lying there; every pore of your body is lifeless.
—*John*

———

Tell your doctor if you're experiencing unrelenting fatigue. The cause could be radiation therapy, but it might also be anemia—especially if you're also having chemotherapy. If so, there are effective treatments (see page 206). Yet another possible reason for fatigue is tumor growth.

Here are a few suggestions for dealing with fatigue; also see Chapter 16.

- Be patient with yourself. Adjust your schedule to diminished energy.

- Nap as needed—and include nap time in your daily schedule.

- Stay as active as possible. You'll feel less fatigued if you exercise regularly.

- Accept offers of help for tiring chores like shopping or housework. But try to remain as involved as possible in enjoyable activities.

Soreness When Swallowing

Radiation to the chest can cause *esophagitis*—inflammation of the esophagus (the tube that connects your throat to your stomach). Though the symptoms come from the esophagus, esophagitis may feel like a sore throat or heartburn: you may experience pain or difficulty swallowing; food may seem to stick in your throat. This is a common problem when radiation is given to the center of the chest.

Report any symptoms to your doctor or radiation nurse, who can evaluate them and provide medication to relieve the problem. Esophagitis is not merely unpleasant; it can lead to malnutrition and weight loss. Also, the same symptoms might be caused by something other than radiation therapy. For example, you might have a fungal infection, such as candidiasis, which requires treatment with antifungal medication.

When esophagitis occurs, it begins a few days to a few weeks after treatment starts. Fortunately, the effects are usually temporary. You should see improvements within two weeks after your treatment ends. For most people, the problem is completely gone after another two weeks to a month.

It's very important to minimize discomfort so you remain able to eat. Here are a few suggestions:

- Avoid foods and beverages that could irritate sensitive tissues, such as anything hot, spicy, or acidic. Coarse, dry foods, such as crackers or nuts, might also be a problem because they can scratch the lining of the esophagus.

- Chew food very well before swallowing. If eating solid food is too uncomfortable, switch to pureed soups, ice cream, and other soft foods. Get nourishment in liquid form from milkshakes, smoothies (for instance, a blend of protein powder and fruit juice or yogurt), or meal replacement beverages such as Ensure.

- Keep your esophagus lubricated. Drink frequently throughout the day. Some people find that chewing gum or sucking on ice chips or popsicles is helpful.

Skin Irritation

Radiation is likely to affect your skin at the place where rays enter your body. Changes similar to those of a sunburn may appear a few days after external radiation treatment starts: redness, irritation, itching, dryness, and increased sensitivity. Most symptoms gradually disappear within a few weeks after treatment ends. But sometimes skin remains slightly darker, drier, and leathery-looking, and more sensitive to sun than it was before.

Discuss any skin problems with your doctor or radiation nurse. They can recommend special products that will greatly alleviate discomfort. You may have favorite home remedies for skin irritation. *Don't use them without checking first.* This caution applies even to normally safe over-the-counter products like petroleum jelly (Vaseline). That's because some medications, lotions, or powders can interfere with radiation and may be difficult to wash off completely.

Here are suggestions for pampering your skin during radiation therapy:

- Avoid sun exposure, which can further irritate your skin. This precaution should continue after treatment, until skin sensitivity is back to normal.

- Wear loose, soft clothing over the affected area.

- Use a mild soap and lukewarm or cool water for washing; pat yourself dry with a soft towel.

- Don't soak in the bath or take long swims—prolonged exposure to water can cause skin problems during radiation treatment.

- Try to avoid extremes of temperature. Don't use heating pads or cold packs, and stay away from hot tubs and saunas.

If these measures are not sufficient, ask your doctor to recommend a soothing medication, lotion, or powder that doesn't interfere with radiation.

Radiation Recall

Some drugs used for chemotherapy may sensitize the skin to radiation. The skin exposed to the beam may develop particularly severe inflammation, rashes, or sores. This phenomenon is called *radiation recall*. If you previously had chemotherapy, you may experience radiation recall when radiation treatment begins. Or it may happen after radiation therapy if you subsequently begin chemotherapy.

If your treatment plan includes both radiation and chemotherapy, ask your doctors if measures can be taken to avoid the problem. Sometimes it's possible to use a different chemotherapy drug that's less likely to produce this sensitivity. If radiation recall occurs, tell your radiation oncologist and oncology nurse. The same measures we suggested for other skin problems may be helpful.

Aching and Stiffness

After radiation to the chest, you may develop aching and stiffness in the muscles of your chest, shoulders, and back. This is caused by minor damage to tissues from radiation, as well as the resulting scarring.

———

Suddenly, every joint in my body hurt—my elbows, fingers, knees, hips, and worst in my neck and shoulders. That went on for months, but it got better.
—*John*

———

The simple stretching exercises described on pages 179–82 can help prevent (or at least minimize) the problem. You can start them while you're getting treatment. After radiation therapy is finished, water exercises are helpful if you have access to a swimming pool. If chlorine irritates your skin, look for an ozone-treated or saltwater pool. Contact ALCASE (Alliance for Lung Cancer Advocacy, Support, and Education) for information about exercise, including water exercises (800-298-2436; *http://www.alcase.org*).

Effects on Lung Function

When lung tumors are treated with radiation, healthy lung tissue inevitably is affected too. That's because tumors are surrounded by normal tissue; also, you breathe during treatment, which causes slight changes in position that can't always be taken into account when the beam is aimed.

Some people who undergo radiation therapy for tumors in the chest develop *radiation pneumonitis*—inflammation of healthy lung tissue that was affected by radiation. Symptoms may be similar to those of a flu: shortness of breath, coughing, and fever. The problem typically develops one to two months after treatment ends. Tell your doctor, who will check for an infection. If you're suffering from radiation pneumonitis, steroid medications can reduce inflammation and make you feel better. Your doctor may prescribe antibiotics as well as steroids, in case there's an infection too.

Lung tissue may become not merely inflamed from radiation treatment, but scarred. This condition is called *radiation fibrosis*. Symptoms are similar to those of pneumonitis, but they appear later (typically after a year) and are not reversible. Fortunately, with current treatment techniques—especially

---

Protecting Your Scalp

I f you receive radiation to the brain, your scalp may become red, itchy, or flaky. Ask your doctor or radiation nurse what you can do for relief. To prevent or minimize problems, protect your scalp during treatment and for as long as sensitivity persists:

- Limit hair washing to twice a week; use a mild or baby shampoo.

- Don't use potentially irritating products or treatments, such as rollers, hot oil, conditioners, dyes, permanent waves, or hair sprays.

- When you're in the sun, cover your head with a hat or scarf.

---

three-dimensional conformal radiation therapy—the incidence of radiation fibrosis is much lower than in the past.

Hair Loss

Radiation can produce temporary or permanent hair loss in the area being treated. Hair loss may be complete, or hair may just get thinner. The problem usually begins two to four weeks after radiation therapy starts. Men who have radiation to the chest may lose body hair in this area. Hair loss on the head is a common side effect of radiation to the brain.

Your radiation oncologist probably can tell you whether or not you can expect your hair to grow back. If hair loss is temporary, regrowth will begin six to eight weeks after treatment ends. As with chemotherapy-related hair loss, new growth may be a different color or texture from what you had before. See pages 195–99 for suggestions on coping with hair loss.

Eating Problems

Radiation therapy may cause loss of appetite, nausea, or indigestion. In addition, fatigue and esophagitis may interfere with eating. The same measures that help with similar chemotherapy-related problems are useful for radiation side effects too (see pages 199–203). If drinking is easier than eat-

For More Information

Here are resources for additional information about radiation therapy:

- *Radiation Therapy and You: A Guide to Self-Help During Cancer Treatment* is an excellent booklet from the National Cancer Institute about radiation therapy. For a free copy, call 800-4-CANCER; the booklet is available online at *http://www.cancer.gov/ cancerinfo/radiation-therapy-and-you*.

- The American Society for Therapeutic Radiology and Oncology offers a free brochure for patients called *Treating Cancer with Radiation Therapy* (703-502-1550; *http://www.astro.org/patient/ treating_cancer/index.htm*).

- The International Radiosurgery Support Association offers patient-oriented information concerning stereotactic radiosurgery, including a list of sites in the United States that offer this treatment and stories about patients who have undergone the procedure. See *http:www.irsa.org*. Printed information can be ordered by calling 717-260-9808.

ing solid food, select nourishing liquids: meal replacement beverages, pureed soups, milk or yogurt, fruit and vegetable juices.

———

When I had radiation near my liver, I had problems with nausea. I took Zofran an hour before treatment, which helped. But even with the Zofran, by the end of the day the smell of food being prepared was nauseating. Halfway through supper I'd start to feel nauseated and would have to lie down to keep from throwing up. Sometimes I'd feel better and would finish my supper. Or my husband would make a milkshake for me with high-fat ice cream to give me some calories.
—Donna P.

———

Effects on Bone Marrow

The big flat bones of your body—collarbone, pelvis, breastbone, and skull—are major bone marrow producers. As with chemotherapy, radiation treatment that passes through these bones can cause myelosuppression (reduced production of white blood cells, red blood cells, or platelets). Fortunately, with radiation therapy the effects usually are less severe. Your blood count will be monitored during treatment. If necessary, problems can be addressed with the same supportive care measures used to treat chemotherapy-induced myelosuppression (see pages 203–206).

Increased Risk of Cancer

Ironically, one of the long-term side effects of radiation therapy is an increased risk of developing a new cancer at the treated site. This danger is lower now than in the past, thanks to more accurate targeting of radiation and safer doses.

Mental Changes after Radiation to the Brain

Early effects usually are produced by swelling of brain tissue. Your doctor may prescribe steroids to prevent swelling. Possible symptoms include confusion, headache, and nausea. Because these symptoms might also be caused by a brain tumor, let your doctor know about them immediately.

Symptoms may appear later as the result of *radiation necrosis*, accumulated dead tissue from the treated tumor. Unlike other parts of the body, the brain lacks an efficient mechanism for disposing of this debris. Late side effects can include impaired memory, diminished intellect, inability to concentrate, and personality changes. Report symptoms to your doctor promptly. Sometimes radiation necrosis can be treated with steroids and other drugs; in rare cases, surgery may be performed to remove dead tissue from the brain.

Radiation therapy is already used extensively to help patients with advanced lung cancer. We expect its role to increase in treatment of early lung cancer as screening becomes more common. With new technology and techniques, radiation therapy will continue to improve, delivering more effective doses with fewer side effects than in the past.

CHAPTER 14

Getting Access to the Latest Treatments

I was diagnosed three years ago. Between then and last summer I'd had surgery, radiation, and three types of chemotherapy, and I'd been in two clinical trials where I got experimental treatments. My best response so far had been "no new growth"—and that was always followed by "growth."

Last July I started a new experimental drug. Once a week I had to go to a research center in Detroit, which is two hours away from where I live. The first results were inconclusive. I got discouraged, but I continued with the treatment.

At the end of August, I called my doctor to get the latest test results. It was my daughter's first day of kindergarten. The doctor is extremely busy and she hadn't had time to check. She pulled the results and began reading them to me. There had been a 50 percent reduction in my tumors. The doctor became so excited that she dropped the phone and started screaming to people across the room. It was as much of a shock as finding out I had cancer, but an unbelievably wonderful shock. I didn't think this would ever happen for me.

—Tracy

Exciting new cancer treatments make headlines every week. But when you check the whole story, you often learn that these promising approaches are still under investigation and won't be available for years. What if that's too long to wait?

One way to gain early access to treatments of the future is to do what Tracy did: volunteer as a research subject. Surprisingly few patients take advantage of this opportunity. According to the American Society of Clinical Oncology, about 20 percent of adult cancer patients are eligible for clinical studies, but fewer than 5 percent actually enroll.

Becoming a research subject is an especially attractive option if your prognosis with standard therapies is poor. There are risks as well as benefits, but many safeguards are built into the process. This chapter will explain how clinical research works and how to find studies that might help you. We'll also describe other ways to obtain treatments that are not yet widely available.

How Clinical Research Tests New Treatments

Clinical research means studies that involve people. When a new treatment is under investigation, clinical research is the last stage in a long testing process. First come laboratory experiments. If the new treatment is a drug, researchers perform tests on blood or tissue samples; they observe effects on microorganisms or on cells. The next step is animal testing. Only after considerable preliminary research do studies begin with human subjects.

All drugs and medical devices must be approved by the Food and Drug Administration (FDA) before doctors can use them in routine practice. The

A Note on Terminology

The terms "clinical research" and "clinical trial" sometimes are used interchangeably. We prefer to make this distinction:

- *Clinical research* refers to any study involving people rather than animals, microorganisms, or cells.

- *Clinical trial* refers to a study that is part of the three-phase research process required for FDA approval of new treatments.

approval process requires *clinical trials*—a series of studies to determine if the measures are both effective and reasonably safe for people. Clinical trials are performed in three phases.

Phase I Clinical Trials

In the case of new drugs, the purpose of phase I trials is to establish safe dosing and to identify side effects; at this stage, investigators are not trying to learn if the treatment actually works. For example, a phase I trial might assess if a drug should be injected or taken by mouth. Or it might use *dose escalation*—higher and higher doses over time—to see how much can be given safely. Phase I trials typically enroll a small number of patients, as few as a dozen. Participation usually is limited to those with late-stage disease who have no other treatment options. Because investigators are not looking at efficacy, they may not require that participants have a particular kind of cancer.

Joining a phase I trial is a gamble. Though you may be helped by the new treatment, that's not the focus of the trial. In drug trials, the odds that you'll benefit are greater if it's not a brand-new drug but an accepted drug or novel combination of accepted drugs being tested for a new purpose. If the drug seems to help, you may be able to continue using it after the study ends. Also, if the phase I study suggests that a higher dose may be effective as well as safe, you might be able to switch to that dose to see if it works for you.

━━━

You're basically donating your body to be used for their research. Eventually I think we'll find a cure for cancer. If I can be one of the links in that, it would be wonderful. But being in a phase I clinical trial is frightening. I want to know what I'll be facing, but they can't tell you what you'll experience. They've never tried it before, so what can they say—"Here's what happened with the rats."
—*Donna P.*

━━━

Phase II Clinical Trials

Once phase I has established a safe dose, phase II trials make a preliminary effort to see if a treatment works; these trials also gather additional information about side effects. One or more groups of about thirty to forty patients are enrolled. As with phase I trials, participation usually is limited to those with advanced disease who don't have other treatment options. Phase II trials may be specific for lung cancer, but usually not for a particular type of lung cancer.

Because the investigators need to assess efficacy in an objective way, they often require that volunteers have readily measured symptoms or tumors. If you are interested in a particular treatment that's in phase II testing but you don't qualify for the first study you find, look around for another trial. The very same treatment may be tested in several phase II trials with different qualifications.

Phase III Clinical Trials

Once phase II trials show that a treatment is effective, phase III trials are conducted to determine if the new measure is superior to existing treatments. These trials are often specific to lung cancer patients and sometimes even to the type of lung cancer. A larger number of patients—usually in the hundreds—are enrolled. Usually they're assigned at random to receive either the existing standard treatment or the therapy under investigation. (This is called a *randomized clinical trial.*) Ongoing results are monitored. If investigators learn in the middle of the trial that one measure is superior, the study will be halted so everyone can receive the better treatment.

After-Market Studies ("Phase IV" Clinical Trials)

After a new treatment has finished phase III clinical trials and received FDA approval, research may continue. These after-market trials (sometimes called phase IV) might investigate:

- Comparisons of approved treatments to see which is most effective.

- Changes in how a treatment is administered. For instance, a study could learn if less frequent (and more convenient) doses of a drug are just as effective.

- Side effects. By administering the treatment to a larger number of patients, doctors learn more about who is affected by particular problems and what supportive measures are most effective.

- Long-term effects of the treatment.

Will I Get a Placebo?

You may be reluctant to consider clinical research for fear of getting a *placebo*—a look-alike treatment that actually contains no active ingredients. If a study does use placebos, the investigators must tell you about that possibility before you join. However, placebos are seldom part of clinical research for cancer treatment.

Phase I and phase II trials rarely use placebos; everyone receives the measure being tested, though the doses may be different. In phase III trials, one group of patients is randomly selected to receive the new treatment, while other patients are given the best currently available treatment. A placebo might be added to an existing treatment. But it wouldn't be used alone unless there was no accepted treatment option. Patients in phase IV studies receive a standard treatment or a variant. Often the "standard treatment" is not an older therapy but a just-approved measure for which more data are sought.

Other Types of Clinical Research

So far we've talked about clinical research focused on cancer treatment. But you also might benefit from studies that test measures for preventing or diagnosing cancer, as well as methods for supportive care.

Cancer Prevention Studies

These studies focus on lifestyle or chemopreventive measures, such as taking food supplements or medications that might prevent cancer. Unlike treatment research, cancer-prevention studies may test a promising measure by comparing it to a placebo. The measures under investigation are usually known to be safe—otherwise they wouldn't be appropriate for cancer prevention, which involves treating people who are healthy.

Because investigators need to see results as quickly as possible, they usually recruit volunteers who are at high risk for the disease, such as lung cancer survivors or those with a smoking history. If you never smoked and have no

Lung Cancer Screening Trials

The National Cancer Institute is sponsoring two major lung cancer screening trials to see if certain tests can reduce deaths. One study, the National Lung Screening Trial (NLST), is recruiting participants. Also underway is the Prostrate, Lung, Colorectal, and Ovarian Cancer Screening Trial (PLCO), which is looking at tests for several cancers; though enrollment is now closed, data collection continues.

Both projects have troubling features:

• Neither study offers all participants the best opportunity for finding an early cancer. In NLST, half the participants will be chosen at random to be checked by CT—but the rest will receive standard chest x-rays, a less sensitive screening method. In PLCO, half the participants received chest x-rays; the rest received whatever health care measures their own doctors provided, so some weren't screened at all.

• Neither study offers expert follow-up if a test is positive. Instead, the person is referred back to his or her primary care physician. There's a risk of unnecessary diagnostic procedures, and a chance that real problems might be missed.

• Results may become moot or inconclusive as technology advances and as people opt to get CT screening on their own.

Our advice:

• If you're at high risk for lung cancer, consider your options carefully before joining NLST. One option is the International Early Lung Cancer Action Project (for information, see http://www .iecap.org); everyone in this study will be examined by CT scans and will receive expert follow-up if results are positive.

• If you're already a PLCO or NLST participant, you can take other measures to protect your health. If you decide to have CT screening outside the study, be sure to inform the trial investigators. If you've already had x-rays as part of one of these trials, tell the radiologist who performs the CT so that your x-rays can be checked.

other risk factors, you may not be eligible for a lung cancer prevention study. However, you can always adopt the healthy lifestyle measures described in Chapter 6.

Cancer Screening Studies

Screening studies investigate ways to discover cancer at its earliest stages. This is especially important for lung cancer, which usually doesn't produce recognizable symptoms until the disease has advanced. Chapter 5 described studies of CT scans and other lung cancer screening methods currently under investigation; see also box on page 235.

Quality of Life Studies

Yet another focus of clinical research involves drugs and other measures—such as diet, exercise, or support groups—aimed at improving the quality of life for cancer patients. Studies might target treatment side effects such as nausea or fatigue, or they might deal with disease symptoms such as breathlessness or pain.

The Pros and Cons of Participating in Research

When you participate in a clinical study, you help advance medical science. What about personal considerations?

On the Plus Side

- You may gain access to a breakthrough treatment that isn't available any other way. For some lung cancer patients, joining a study has meant the difference between life and death.

- You may be treated or monitored by doctors and other medical personnel with special expertise in lung cancer.

- Part of your treatment may be free; some or all of your treatment-related expenses, such as travel, may be paid for.

Would I Have to Travel? Switch Doctors?

Some cancer patients are willing to travel long distances for promising experimental treatments, but this isn't practical or acceptable for everyone. However, you may be able to participate in a clinical study without leaving your hometown or seeing a new doctor.

Many local hospitals are affiliated with cancer centers or cancer research groups through the National Cancer Institute's Community Clinical Oncology Program (CCOP). This program allows doctors and patients in all parts of the country to participate in clinical research. Even if you enter a study at a cancer center in another community, you probably won't have to change doctors. To make participation as convenient as possible, investigators often minimize out-of-town visits and allow patients' own oncologists to handle most of their care; or they arrange to cover travel expenses for participants.

Potential Disadvantages and Problems

- New treatments may not work well—they might even be inferior to existing measures. Or they may have unexpected side effects.

- If the study is comparing two measures, you won't be able to select the treatment you receive.

- Participation may involve time-consuming obligations, such as extra tests, medical visits, or record keeping. This can be a problem for doctors as well as patients.

- Your insurer may be unwilling to pay for costs that are not covered by the trial's sponsor. For instance, the sponsor may provide the drug but expect you or your insurance company to pay for the nursing care required to administer the drug. (See box on page 244 for suggestions on dealing with your insurer.)

In addition to these general points, each study has its own risks and benefits. The investigators or clinical trial nurse will explain them in detail before you join, as we'll describe below.

How to Find Studies

The first step is to talk to your doctor, who may know about—or be willing to help you locate—useful studies. But even a lung cancer specialist may not be aware of every investigation that might be helpful to you. So it's best to search for yourself too.

Unfortunately, there's no single listing of all clinical research opportunities. Below are resources to check. If you have Internet access, the easiest way to cover all these resources is to work your way through the list of links about clinical trials at Lung Cancer Online (*http://www.lungcanceronline.org/ treatment-experimental/clinicaltrials.html*). Especially valuable are Lung Cancer Online's links to individual cancer centers and drug companies, whose web sites may describe studies that aren't listed elsewhere.

National Cancer Institute (NCI)

NCI maintains the PDQ (Physician Data Query) database, one of the most comprehensive listings of clinical studies. Call its Cancer Information Service, 800-4-CANCER, to ask for a customized search of the database; your physician can request a customized search on your behalf by calling 800-345-3300. Or you can access the database directly online at *http:// www.cancer.gov/search/clinicaltrials/usersguides*. Also check NCI's excellent general information about clinical trials at *http://cancertrials.nci.nih.gov*.

CenterWatch

CenterWatch is a publisher whose specialty is clinical trials. Its web site—*http://www.centerwatch.com*—contains helpful articles and other information about clinical trials. You can search the site for industry- and government-funded studies that are looking for participants. CenterWatch also offers a free e-mail service that notifies you of any new trials for which you might be eligible. If you don't have Internet access, you can request information by calling CenterWatch at 617-856-5900 and asking for the Internet Services Department.

Food and Drug Administration (FDA)

The FDA's Cancer Liaison Program web site (*http://www.fda.gov/oashi/ cancer/cancer.html*) contains information about clinical trials. You can also contact the Cancer Liaison Program via the FDA's Office of Special Issues at 301-827-4460.

ALCASE (Alliance for Lung Cancer Advocacy, Support, and Education)

The ALCASE web site (*http://www.alcase.org*) has useful general articles about clinical research, and sometimes offers information about specific studies. Or call 800-298-2436 to talk to a counselor about clinical trials.

Cancer Care

Cancer Care's web site has a very informative section about clinical trials for cancer (*http://www.cancercare.org/ClinicalTrials/ClinicalTrialsMain.cfm*), including a useful list of links for additional information. You can sign up for Cancer Care's free e-mail newsletter, called *Clinical Trials E-Update*.

Individual Cancer Centers and Other Medical Centers

Many hospitals and medical schools recruit patients for clinical research. Not all of these studies are included in the comprehensive listings mentioned above, but they can be tracked down via each institution.

Start with nearby cancer centers and teaching hospitals. Check their web sites, which may list clinical studies. You can also telephone the institution and ask for its office for clinical research. Explain your situation and ask if you're eligible for any studies that are seeking volunteers.

To broaden your search to other geographical areas, try the following:

- The National Cancer Institute's list of designated cancer centers—leading medical centers that specialize in cancer—is posted on the NCI web site (*http://www.nci.nih.gov/cancercenters/centerslist.html*); you can also call 800-4-CANCER (800-422-6237) for information about the centers.

- Lung Cancer Online offers a list of links, organized by state, to the web sites of leading lung cancer centers (*http://www.lungcanceronline.org/care-programs/index.html*).

Drug Companies

Pharmaceutical companies sponsor clinical research on both new and established products. Many, but not all, of these studies are listed by the National Cancer Institute. If you're interested in a particular drug, check the information posted on the manufacturer's web site. Lung Cancer Online has a comprehensive list of links to pharmaceutical companies (*http://www.lung canceronline.org/sites/pharmcos.html*). Or call the company to ask about research opportunities. To obtain manufacturers' telephone numbers, try toll-free directory assistance (800-555-1212) or check the *Physicians' Desk Reference* at your local library.

The Patient Grapevine

If you belong to a patient support group or keep in touch with other lung cancer survivors online, you may get leads to new studies that are looking for volunteers. Marcel Baruch—who is battling stage IV disease—described how he learned about a promising clinical trial:

> *I belong to a Cancer Care support group. One of the ladies was telling us about a clinical trial she was in at Sloan-Kettering with a medicine called Iressa. She had been taking the medicine for a year and she felt terrific. They weren't accepting any more patients for this trial, but one day she mentioned to me that a friend had told her about a trial with a similar drug that New York University had started. I entered the trial.*

Deciding If a Study Is Right for You

Once you've identified clinical studies of possible interest, you'll need to learn more about them. Not all studies are appropriate or desirable for all patients.

Talk to Your Doctor

The first step is to discuss the study with your oncologist or primary care physician. If your doctor recommends against it, ask why—and listen

If You're Interested in Joining a Clinical Study

To maximize your chances of qualifying for a study, start looking as soon as possible. Some projects accept patients only if they are **treatment-naive** (haven't yet been treated at all) or if they have recently undergone lung cancer surgery or other specified treatment.

Before you begin your search, gather the information below. That way you'll know which projects might be appropriate, and you'll be able to answer investigators' preliminary questions:

- Type and stage of your cancer

- Treatments you've already received, dates of treatment, and the names of any drugs you've been given

- Your progress to date

This may sound daunting, but most of the information is in your medical records. Your doctor can fill in any missing pieces. Ask a friend to help if you feel overwhelmed. Updates will be much easier.

carefully to the reasons. The concerns could be legitimate. For example, the experimental treatment may entail risks you haven't considered. Perhaps the standard treatment is very effective so there's little to gain by trying something else. On the other hand, the doctor's objections might involve less relevant issues such as extra record keeping. To help clarify any uncertainties, arrange for your doctor to speak with the physician in charge of the research.

———

At first I looked for any trials. I came up with a lot of crazy things. I'd bring them to my doctor and then struggle to understand while he explained why they weren't appropriate. Now I'm more careful.
—Tracy

———

Are You Eligible?

All studies have eligibility requirements. Investigators may limit participation to those most likely to be helped (or least likely to be harmed). They
may want to eliminate factors that might confuse the results, such as certain
previous treatments. Sometimes they need participants for whom the effects
of treatment will be easy to assess; that's why some studies are open only to
volunteers whose tumors are measurable. Listings of clinical studies include
brief descriptions of their eligibility criteria. If you call an investigator to learn
more about a particular project, you may hear about further requirements.

Safeguards for Patients

Clinical research always includes safeguards for participating patients.
Investigators must submit their research plans to the **Institutional Review
Board** (IRB) at their hospital, university, or other study site. The IRB, whose
members include lay people as well as scientists and health professionals, reviews
proposed studies to make sure patients won't be exposed to inappropriate risks.

Another safeguard is the **informed consent** process. Before you join, the
investigators will tell you what the study will entail, including all the potential risks and benefits. You'll be given a detailed written summary and asked
to sign a form indicating that you understand the information and agree to
participate. Read the consent form very carefully. Don't hesitate to ask questions if something isn't clear.

Even after you've been through the informed consent procedure and
have joined a trial, you still have the right to withdraw at any time. During the
study, the investigators will monitor your response to treatment. If there's any
evidence of harm, or if another measure is found to be more effective, your
treatment will be stopped so that you can receive the best available therapy.

---

*I volunteered for a phase I antibody trial. They gave me an injection
of an antibody to attack the cancer. It didn't work. My blood pressure
got dangerously low even though I was on a low dose and they were
pumping fluids into me. They kicked me out of the trial. At the time
you think, "Why are you kicking me out? Give me the drug!" But I
needed to be out of that trial.*
—Tracy

Blinding

Expectation—both the patient's and the doctor's—can affect research results. To prevent bias about efficacy or side effects, studies may be blinded. This can be done in two different ways:

- *Single-blind study:* The patients don't know which treatment they're receiving, but the doctors do.

- *Double-blind study:* Neither the investigators nor the patients know who is getting which treatment.

When a study is double-blind, ongoing results are monitored by researchers who are not directly involved in data collection. If one treatment proves to be much better than the other, the study will be stopped so that everyone can receive the superior treatment.

Questions to Ask Before Joining a Study

The informed consent process provides an excellent opportunity for you to address your concerns. Write down your questions in advance. Since it's difficult to absorb all the information, we suggest that you take notes, make an audio recording of the meeting, or ask a close friend or relative to accompany you. Here are some issues you might want to discuss:

Background Information

Ask about the purpose of the research and who is sponsoring it. Find out about previous studies of the experimental treatment. How many people have received it? What were the results? Insist on hearing the bad news as well as the promising findings. For instance, how many patients have had to drop out of the study, and why?

Study Design

Ask the investigators to explain their plans for investigating the new treatment. Will different treatments be given to different groups? If so, will you know which treatment you receive?

What about Insurance?

Some insurance companies and HMOs provide full or partial coverage when patients join a clinical trial; others do not. Because clinical research is so important, Congress is considering action that would improve insurance coverage for treatments under investigation. Meanwhile, your doctor and the research team may be able to negotiate an arrangement with your insurer. Often they can make the convincing argument that it's less expensive for you to be treated in the study. Some cancer patients are so eager to participate in research that they lay out money themselves, and later battle their insurance company—sometimes successfully—for reimbursement.

For more information, see the National Cancer Institute's free booklet *Clinical Trials and Insurance Coverage: A Resource Guide* (800-4-CANCER; *http://www.cancer.gov/clinicaltrials/understanding/insurance-coverage*.

What to Expect

Learn about the details of treatment—where it takes place and on what schedule. Find out what tests and other procedures you will receive. Will any of them be painful or unpleasant? What will be done to relieve any side effects?

Risks and Benefits

During the informed consent process, you'll learn about the expected risks and benefits of treatment. Also discuss your other treatment options, including the possibility of participating in a different study.

Expenses

Ask about your out-of-pocket expenses, if any. Some studies cover not only medical but also nonmedical expenses, such as travel or child care. Inquire about the possibility of getting insurance coverage.

After the Study Is Over

Find out if the study involves any long-term follow-up. Ask if you can continue the treatment after the study ends.

Other Ways to Obtain Experimental Treatments

You may learn about a promising drug that's under investigation, but be unable or unwilling to participate in a clinical study that's testing it. Maybe you don't meet the eligibility requirements; perhaps the location makes it impossible. If it's a phase III study, maybe you don't want to take the chance that you'll be randomly assigned to the standard treatment. Here are other options:

Compassionate Use

If you are seriously ill, your doctor may be able to obtain the drug for you under the Food and Drug Administration's *compassionate use* guidelines, which is also called emergency use or *single-patient IND (Investigational New Drug)*. This procedure shortcuts the long testing process for new drugs, but still retains safeguards for patients. Because of these safeguards— and because one purpose of the guidelines is to obtain additional data on new drugs' safety and effectiveness—extra paperwork is required. If you want to participate, here's what your doctor must do:

- Obtain a letter from the manufacturer granting permission to use the drug and agreeing to provide it. Some manufacturers do this routinely; others may be reluctant to send the drug to a single patient and monitor the results. Even if they're eager to help, they may not have a sufficient supply to meet requests from individuals, especially in early stages of product development when manufacturing facilities are not set up.

- Write a treatment plan and an informed consent statement, and arrange for them to be approved by the appropriate Institutional Review Board (IRB).

- Submit an application to the FDA, including a required form, your medical history, a summary of the doctor's qualifications, and all the supporting material mentioned above (letter from the drug company, treatment plan, signed informed consent form, IRB approval).

- Contact the drug manufacturer after the FDA approves compassionate use, so that a supply can be sent.

- During and after treatment, submit data on any side effects or changes in your condition.

For information and instructions, including a link to the necessary form, see the FDA's web page titled "Access to Unapproved Drugs" (*http://www.fda.gov/cder/cancer/access.htm*); or call the FDA's Office of Special Health Issues at 301-827-4460.

Off-Label Treatment

Sometimes a new lung cancer treatment involves a drug or a combination of drugs that have already received FDA approval for another purpose—such as treating a different form of cancer. It's legal for your doctor to prescribe any FDA-approved drug, even for a use that is not specifically approved. Some doctors are willing to provide off-label treatment; others are reluctant to do so. Also, not all insurers will cover off-label treatment, even if it is approved by a doctor, so check first.

Foreign Sources

New drugs that are still at the testing stage in the United States may already be on the market in other countries. Some cancer patients travel outside the United States to buy such drugs or to be treated with them; others obtain these medications by mail.

Be aware that it's not legal to import drugs that are not FDA-approved. However, the FDA's enforcement guidelines suggest "a more permissive policy" under certain circumstances: if quantities are small (e.g., a three-month supply for one person) and if the drug will be used under the supervision of a licensed doctor for a serious condition for which other effective treatment is not available. The purposes of these guidelines are to conserve enforcement resources and to accommodate individuals who have no other treatment options. Note, however, that the guidelines are merely suggestions; importing nonapproved drugs is against the law and may not be permitted by an individual FDA enforcement agent, even if the patient meets the standards.

If you are thinking about purchasing unapproved cancer drugs abroad, get current information on the FDA's policies and enforcement guidelines. Read the FDA's warning about purchasing medication outside the United States (*http://www.fda.gov/ora/import/purchasing_medications.htm*), where drugs may not be subject to rigorous testing and manufacturing controls to assure safety and efficacy. Also see the FDA's detailed information about enforcement guidelines (*http://www.fda.gov/ora/import/pipinfo.htm*). The same information can be obtained from the FDA's toll-free information line: 888-INFO-FDA.

Tracy's tumors, which decreased dramatically the first month after she began an experimental treatment, showed a further reduction a month later. At that point, the disease stabilized. But the tumors were 80 percent smaller than when she started. Tracy reports:

> *I have CT scans every other month. The drug's side effects are
> minimal, mostly a rash and dry skin that doesn't heal well. I'll take it
> until the disease progresses or I have serious side effects.*

We urge every lung cancer patient—and every physician who treats lung cancer patients—to consider clinical research. New and improved treatments for this disease will emerge only through these investigations. Yet studies sometimes move more slowly than they might because investigators can't find all the participants they need. The benefits are personal, too. Your options expand if you include experimental as well as standard treatments. And you just might find something that really works.

CHAPTER 15

Complementary and Alternative Therapies

Chemotherapy was terribly hard on me. I became weak. I developed awful gastrointestinal problems; I had so much pain in my legs that some days I couldn't even put my feet on the ground. I didn't want to pour more poison into my body. I was willing to look at new things, because I know that traditional Western medicine doesn't have all the answers.

—*Joyce*

E ven if you're under the care of excellent doctors, you probably will ask yourself: What else can I do? Your quest may lead you to try (or at least consider) alternative and complementary therapies—measures that are not part of standard Western medicine. If so, you're not alone. Surveys indicate that nearly half of Americans use these treatments, and the proportion is even higher for people with cancer.

In a study of 453 patients at the M. D. Anderson Cancer Center in Texas, 83 percent reported that they'd used at least one complementary or alternative therapy. Measures included prayer, herbs and vitamins, exercise, massage, folk remedies, and various products touted as cancer cures.

Why would these people—all of whom were receiving care at one of America's leading cancer centers—turn to nonstandard treatments? According to the study, which was published in 2000 in the *Journal of Clinical Oncology*, the most common reason was a desire to feel hopeful. This and other surveys suggest that patients usually are seeking to expand their options rather than to abandon mainstream medicine. They see these measures as more natural and less invasive additions that can enhance wellness, relieve symptoms, and make them feel better.

Some CAM (complementary and alternative medicine) therapies are valuable and safe. But others may be useless or even risky. This book can't possibly cover everything that's available. However, we'll tell you about a few methods that cancer experts agree are worthwhile. None promises a cure, but all are valuable complements to conventional treatment. We'll also give you resources for exploring further.

We hope you will be open to the possibilities. However, we want to emphasize that unproven therapies should never substitute for conventional medical care.

Before you try any CAM therapy, discuss it with your doctor.
Tell your medical caregivers about all the CAM treatments you use.

A Note on Terminology

The terms "complementary" and "alternative" mean different things to different people, so you may have seen them explained in different ways. In this book, we follow the definitions used by the National Cancer Institute.

Complementary and alternative medicine, abbreviated *CAM*, refers to a very wide range of healing approaches that have not traditionally been part of conventional medical treatment in the United States. A particular CAM measure could be considered complementary or alternative, depending on whether the patient also seeks conventional treatment:

- *Complementary therapies* are used *in addition to* conventional treatment.

- *Alternative therapies* are used *instead of* conventional treatment (something we do *not* recommend).

Mainstream Medicine
Takes a Closer Look

A landmark Harvard survey, published in the prestigious *New England Journal of Medicine* in 1993, startled the medical establishment with its finding that one American in three used nonstandard approaches. The medical community has responded with a blend of interest and caution.

Growing Acceptance

Physicians, who until recently might have dismissed CAM treatments as quackery, are becoming more open to them—at least as complements to conventional cancer care. Leading cancer centers and teaching hospitals have adopted certain complementary therapies, such as acupuncture and massage. This approach is sometimes called ***integrative medicine.*** In a survey published in the *Journal of the American Medical Association* in 1998, 75 of the 125 medical schools in the United States reported that they offer courses on complementary therapies or include them in required courses.

In 1992 the National Institutes of Health established the Office of Alternative Medicine (OAM) to coordinate research efforts on non-standard medicine. This effort was greatly expanded in 1998. OAM was upgraded from an office to a center, becoming the National Center for Complementary and Alternative Medicine (NCCAM); its annual budget leaped from about $2 million to nearly $70 million. NCCAM conducts and supports clinical research on a wide range of nonconventional therapies. Their cancer-related studies include investigations of a promising shark cartilage extract (now in phase III clinical trials cosponsored by the National Cancer Institute) and a controversial alternative therapy featuring coffee enemas.

Remaining Doubts

Despite increased acceptance of CAM, many doctors still have significant reservations about these therapies—and not without reason. Though some approaches have been evaluated by scientific studies, these treatments have not been through the clinical trial system (described in Chapter 14). Nor are they subject to the safeguards that protect consumers from incompetent traditional medical practitioners and unsafe drugs.

All physicians must be licensed by their state to practice medicine. In contrast, only some alternative practitioners are state-licensed. Unlicensed (and licensed) practitioners may be certified by their own professional organizations, but others operate without such oversight.

Similarly, dietary supplements and herbal remedies sold as dietary supplements (as most are) are not regulated nearly as strictly as drugs are. Under the provisions of the Dietary Supplement Health and Education Act of 1994 (DSHEA), manufacturers must make sure that the product is safe and that label information is truthful. However, the Food and Drug Administration does not review these products to assure that manufacturers have actually produced a safe product with a truthful label, as it does with drugs. Only if a supplement is found to be unsafe can the FDA stop its sale.

Supplements, like all consumer products, also are regulated by the Federal Trade Commission (FTC), which requires that advertising be truthful and not misleading. When products make health claims, the FTC typically uses FDA findings to determine if the claims are acceptable. (See box below on reading product labels.)

Physicians fear that a patient might substitute an unproven alternative therapy for a conventional treatment that can prolong survival, reduce symptoms, or even cure the disease. They also worry that some people with cancer, who already are financially pressed, may pay hundreds or even thousands of dollars for worthless treatments.

Another concern—one that deserves more attention from doctors—is that alternative therapies can interfere with conventional treatment. In the previously mentioned survey of M. D. Anderson cancer patients, an alarming

Read the Label

Certain FDA-approved health claims, which are supported by scientific evidence, may be included on the label of a product sold as a dietary supplement. If any other claims are made, the following also must appear: *"This statement has not been evaluated by the Food and Drug Administration. This product is not intended to diagnose, treat, cure, or prevent any disease."*

Does CAM Distort Research Findings?

The "Don't ask, don't tell" approach to CAM not only endangers patients. It also compromises research on conventional treatments. We know from careful surveys that most cancer patients use nonstandard therapies and that they usually don't tell their doctors. Yet investigators rarely question research volunteers about their use of CAM.

Even such common measures as vitamin supplements can affect cancer treatment outcomes. Until researchers ask appropriately detailed questions about CAM, we won't know if cancer study findings have been distorted by therapies that patients haven't mentioned or been asked about.

65 percent of these who were using CAM didn't tell their oncologists, and in most cases their doctors didn't ask. This failure to communicate puts patients at risk for dangerous—even deadly—interactions between their conventional treatments and their undisclosed CAM measures. Here are just a few examples:

- Vitamins A, C, and E protect the body against oxidation, a process that can damage the DNA of cells. But antioxidants may interfere with the effects of chemotherapy and radiation, which deliberately damage cancerous cells.

- Vitamin K, which promotes blood clotting, can interfere with medications that intentionally inhibit clotting (blood thinners). Many people with lung cancer take these drugs to prevent life-threatening clots that could cause a *pulmonary embolism* (blood clot in the lungs), a heart attack, or a stroke. Herbal products that contain vitamin K, such as blue-green algae, could have similar adverse effects on these individuals.

- St. John's wort, taken for depression and anxiety, may intensify the effects of certain anesthetics and painkillers. This could cause problems during and after surgery.

- Ginkgo biloba, used to improve memory and blood circulation, can impair blood clotting, thereby increasing the risks of surgery and other procedures that cause bleeding.

- A very strict low-fat vegetarian diet, which may be acceptable and even beneficial for some individuals, might endanger someone already weakened by cancer-related weight loss.

Making the Most of the Mind-Body Connection

We all know from everyday experience that our minds can affect our bodies. Our heart races during a scary movie; a stressful day can leave us with a throbbing headache. Without thinking of yourself as a New Age healer, you've probably devised simple mental strategies for dealing with physical problems. Perhaps you take slow, deep breaths to ease tension, or you deliberately distract yourself to counter pain.

CAM offers a variety of techniques that can help you channel the power of your mind to help your body. These methods have gained wide acceptance among conventional practitioners because of strong scientific evidence that they're safe and effective. They can help you relax and improve your mood; they may also be effective against pain and nausea. There's even some evidence—though it's controversial—that by reducing stress, mind-body techniques enhance the immune system, which helps to prevent or fight cancer.

Treatments that improve your quality of life can produce real improvements in your health as well. We encourage you to consider the methods described below and to discuss them with your doctor.

Support Groups

In the 1970s, Stanford University psychiatrist David Spiegel and colleagues randomly assigned eighty-six women with advanced breast cancer to two groups. All received standard medical care, but half also attended weekly support group meetings. At the end of each meeting, participants practiced a simple self-hypnosis exercise aimed at helping them deal with pain. Before the study began and at four-month intervals, the researchers questioned the women about their symptoms and their mood.

After a year, the women who had received only standard care showed increases in negative emotions: they were more anxious and depressed; they also felt more fatigued. In contrast, the mood of those who participated in

Lessons from the Placebo Effect

Scientific studies of medical treatments sometimes compare the measure being tested to a placebo—a look-alike pill or procedure with no known medical value. The placebo might be a pill that contains only sugar or starch, or fake acupuncture in which needles are inserted into spots other than the designated points on the body used by real acupuncturists. Almost always, some patients who receive placebos show improvements. Indeed, some studies find the placebo is just as helpful as the "real" treatment.

One reason for the placebo effect is that many conditions improve without any intervention. A Danish study published in the *New England Journal of Medicine* in 2001, which examined studies whose experimental design included both placebo and "no treatment" groups, found no difference between the two when treatment outcomes could be measured objectively. Does this mean that the placebo effect doesn't really exist? No. In studies where the outcomes were subjective—for example, in investigations of pain—those who were given placebos generally reported more benefit than those who received no treatment.

The placebo effect shows the power of hope and the value of positive emotions in medicine. Negative thinking is powerful too—but in the other direction. That's one reason some doctors are reluctant to warn patients about possible treatment side effects. When bad thoughts produce harmful consequences for health, it's called a *nocebo effect*.

support groups had actually improved. They were less anxious, less depressed, and less exhausted. Moreover, they reported significantly less pain than women in the control group.

But the most dramatic benefit wasn't revealed until ten years later, when investigators traced the study participants to find out what had happened to them. All but three of the women had died. That wasn't surprising, since all had advanced disease. However, the average survival time was nearly twice as long for those who had been in support groups—37 months compared to 19

Breathing Away Stress

Here's a simple technique that not only counters stress but also gives your respiratory muscles a mini-workout. Combine belly breathing (see pages 28–29) with *pursed-lip breathing*—exhaling through pursed lips, as if you were blowing out a candle or whistling, but without sound. Pursed-lip breathing exercises the muscles used to exhale because it requires them to work a little harder.

- Inhale slowly through your nose. Your diaphragm will relax and your abdomen will push out. Count slowly as you inhale. Over time, try to make your inhalations longer, so you fill your lungs more completely.

- Exhale through pursed lips, pulling in your abdomen to squeeze as much air as possible out of your lungs. Though your lips should provide resistance, they should be open enough so that breathing is not labored. Count slowly as you exhale. Take twice as long to exhale as you did to inhale.

- Pause for a few seconds, so you don't hyperventilate and become light-headed. Then repeat.

While you're learning the technique, do the breathing exercise while lying on a bed or on the floor. Afterward, you can combine it with other activities. For instance you can practice belly and pursed-lip breathing while walking or watching television—or any time you want to reduce stress.

months for those who received only standard care. Furthermore, all three of the ten-year survivors had been in support groups.

The impact of support groups seems almost miraculous, but there are rational explanations. Support and encouragement improve mood. If patients are happier and their pain is under control, they're likely to sleep and eat better—which makes them feel healthier; cancer treatment seems more tolerable and is less likely to be discontinued. (For information on finding support groups, see page 137.)

Meditation

Meditation is a mental and physical relaxation technique that has long been part of religious practice. Research confirms that it has impressive physical and mental benefits, including lowering blood pressure, reducing stress, and countering chronic pain and insomnia.

Your hospital may offer instruction in meditation; if not, your medical team may be able to refer you to a class or instructor. Local community centers, adult education programs, or health clubs may offer classes. Some lung cancer survivors benefit from exercise with components that include meditation and relaxation, such as qi gong, tai chi, and yoga. Check with your doctor before you start any exercise program, and be sure to tell the instructor that you are a lung cancer survivor. For more information about meditation, including instructions, see Dr. Herbert Benson's classic book *The Relaxation Response*, recently updated and expanded (Wholecare, 2000).

Hypnosis

Hypnosis and self-hypnosis combine deep relaxation and focused attention to particular goals or ideas. A 1995 National Institutes of Health consensus development panel found that hypnosis can relieve pain. Other research suggests that it counters nausea and vomiting for some people. Portrayals of hypnosis in the popular media can be misleading. You don't lose consciousness; you're not in a trance; you can't be manipulated against your will. Rather, being under hypnosis is like engrossing yourself in a book: you don't pay attention to the casual conversations around you and you might not notice that you're getting hungry—but you'd certainly respond to a fire alarm. See the box on the next page for instructions.

Imagery

Imagery is simply using the imagination to visualize helpful or distracting pictures. For example, if you're tense before or during a medical procedure, you might relax by picturing yourself floating in a peaceful lake. Some patients imagine video games in which cancer cells are gobbled up or exploded. Imagery may be guided: an instructor, who may be present or on a tape, describes the scenes.

A Technique for Self-Hypnosis

Before you start, decide what you want to work on. For instance, if you're suffering from pain or nausea, you could focus on clearing away the problem and feeling better. Use the following relaxation technique or any other method that works for you:

- Sit or lie in a quiet place where you can be warm and comfortable.

- Close your eyes and relax.

- Imagine yourself slowly descending a staircase into a dark room. Very slowly, count backward from ten to one. Take one to three minutes to complete the count. With each number, imagine yourself descending the staircase and becoming more relaxed. If you become distracted (which is normal when you're learning the technique), simply start over.

- When you reach zero, the bottom of the staircase, you will feel very relaxed and very light. You'll have a sense of isolation and detachment from your surroundings, as if you were in a capsule—though you can hear and see if you need to. With practice, you'll be able to reach this stage more easily and smoothly.

- Focus on the planned topic for as long as you wish, from a few minutes to half an hour or longer.

- When you're finished, sit or lie quietly for a few minutes, allowing your attention to return to normal.

Studies suggest that imagery can help manage pain and nausea, as well as anxiety and stress. To learn more, talk to your oncology team; they may be able to recommend a psychologist or other professional who can teach you the technique. Or read *Getting Well Again*, by Dr. O. Carl Simonton and Stephanie Mathews-Simonton (Bantam, 1992), who pioneered this treatment for cancer patients.

Prayer and Spirituality

Whatever your beliefs, you can benefit from spending time in contemplation and asking for help from God, the collective consciousness, the universe, or any higher power that resonates with you. You don't need to be a member of any particular religion or even have religious faith. Research finds that virtually any type of prayer and spirituality can reduce stress, anxiety, and depression and enhance well-being.

A religious or spiritual adviser, if you have one, can offer suggestions. One popular book on prayer and medicine that is recommended by many cancer patients is *Healing Words: The Power of Prayer and the Practice of Medicine*, by Larry Dossey, M.D. (HarperSanFrancisco, 1993).

———

I'm a pretty religious person. I've used two Bible verses as meditation techniques. One is "Be still, and know that I am God." When I'm anxious, I repeat that over and over. I hate MRIs. When I'm having one, the verse helps quiet the anxious wanderings of my mind.

Praying for Miracles

*P*eople *who pray for miracles usually don't get miracles, any more than children who pray for bicycles, good grades, or boyfriends get them as a result of praying. But people who pray for courage, for strength to bear the unbearable, for the grace to remember what they have left instead of what they have lost, very often find their prayers answered. They discover that they have more strength, more courage than they ever knew themselves to have. Where did they get it? I would like to think that their prayers helped them find that strength. Their prayers helped them tap hidden reserves of faith and courage that were not available to them before.*

—Rabbi Harold S. Kushner

Quoted by permission from *When Bad Things Happen to Good People*, by Rabbi Harold S. Kushner (Avon, 1994)

The other verse is "God will not forget you. He has your image carved in the palm of His hand." This is comforting when I'm on a cold table for a test or treatment and feeling defenseless. I believe that God cares for me. Repeating the words helps me remember that and not feel alone, like a broken and discarded thing.
—*Tracy*

Other Mind-Body Measures

The techniques described above are just a few of the measures that can help cancer patients improve their mood and quality of life. Find out what's offered at your hospital; talk to your medical team and to other patients. Possibilities include journal keeping, art or music therapy, and even humor therapy.

Symptom Relief from Hands-On Treatments

Some CAM methods involve touching or manipulating the body. Like the mind-body techniques, they can reduce stress and improve mood. Some can also relieve physical symptoms and side effects, including pain, nausea, and vomiting. Discuss these measures with your doctor before you start. Though they're generally safe and effective, there could be reasons not to use them, especially during your medical treatment.

Acupuncture and Acupressure

Acupuncture is an ancient Chinese medical technique in which fine, flexible needles are inserted into particular points on the body that are believed to correspond to different organs. A consensus panel of medical experts convened by the National Institutes of Health, which conducted an exhaustive review of the medical literature, concluded in 1997 that acupuncture treatment is effective for the nausea and vomiting of chemotherapy. Many patients find that acupuncture also is helpful against pain, and that its side effects are much milder than those of painkilling medication.

▬

*The first time I had acupuncture was before the lung cancer. I'd had
terrible shoulder pain. I was a little afraid of the needles, but I
decided to try it because the painkiller and the muscle relaxant
weren't helping. The needles weren't a problem—it's not like getting
injections. After eight sessions, the pain went away.*

*I felt so sick from the chemotherapy that I called my insurance
company to find out where I could go for acupuncture. I was sent to
the pain clinic at the hospital. An oncology nurse there gives me
acupuncture under the direction of an M.D. She's a licensed
acupuncturist and knows a lot about Chinese medicine. I've been
going every week. I think it has helped some with the neuropathy and
stress. But you can't cut me in half to find out. The same nurse also
tried working with me on my gastrointestinal problems but it didn't
help much.*

—Joyce

▬

Acupressure is similar to acupuncture, but uses pressure instead of needles. Two variants are shiatsu and tuina, in which acupuncture points are
stimulated by massage.

Talk to your doctor before you undergo acupuncture or acupressure
treatment, so you can be sure it's safe. For example, acupuncture is not
appropriate for anyone suffering from myelosuppression (reduced bone
marrow activity): if white blood cell counts are low, there's an increased risk
of infection; if the platelet count is low, there's an increased risk of bleeding.
For added safety, make sure the therapist you choose uses disposable needles.
And be sure to explain that you're a lung cancer survivor.

Many cancer centers and hospitals now offer acupuncture. Ask your
doctor or oncology nurse to refer you to a qualified acupuncturist. Select a
licensed practitioner if your state has a licensing program (most do). The
National Certification Commission for Acupuncture and Oriental Medicine
(NCCAOM) certifies acupuncturists. Its web site (*http://www.nccaom.org*)
has information and a searchable directory; or call 703-548-9004.

For more information about acupuncture, see the excellent article from
the National Center for Complementary and Alternative Medicine, available
online (*http://nccam.nih.gov/health/acupuncture*) or from the NCCAM
Clearinghouse (888-644-6226).

For Relief of Nausea

Several controlled studies have found that pressure to a particular point on the forearm combats nausea and vomiting. Pressure can be applied by fingers or by beads that are held against special points on the wrist by elasticized bands. Though the bands are available at drugstores and are convenient to use, they may not exert sufficient pressure. To use your fingers:

• Hold one arm out in front of you with the palm up. Locate the nausea pressure point by placing the middle three fingers of the other hand across the wrist, with the ring finger at the crease. The point is 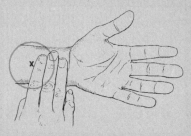 just after the index finger in the center of your forearm, between the two tendons you can feel through your skin.

• Using your thumb, place firm (but not uncomfortable) pressure on the point. It may take up to five minutes to experience relief.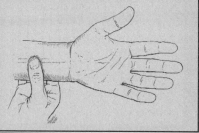

Massage

Massage—stroking, rubbing, or kneading the soft tissues of the body— promotes muscle relaxation, which contributes to both physical and emotional well-being. Research suggests that massage can relieve pain (which is often caused or exacerbated by muscle tension), reduce stress and anxiety, and improve mood. Because of these benefits, some cancer centers and hospitals now offer massage to patients.

Talk to your doctor or oncology nurse to make sure that massage is safe for you. For example, it may not be appropriate during radiation treatment because of skin sensitivity. Massage is performed in many different ways, from the light touch of reiki (in which the practitioner may not actually touch the patient) to the deep manipulation of Rolfing. Vigorous versions are not advised for areas of the body affected by cancer or cancer treatment.

Your medical team may be able to refer you to a massage therapist. Practitioners are licensed in just over half the states in the United States. The National Certification Board for Therapeutic Massage and Bodywork certifies massage therapists and can provide referrals (800-296-0664 or 703-610-9015; *http://www.ncbtmb.com*). For more information about a wide variety of healing massage techniques, contact the American Massage Therapy Association (847-864-0123; *http://www.amtamassage.org*). If you decide to schedule a massage, tell the therapist that you are being treated for lung cancer.

Investigating Other CAM Therapies

The measures described above are just a few of the possibilities. To learn more, start with the resources below; they present useful general guidance, as well as information about specific treatments. As we've emphasized, it's very important to discuss CAM treatments with your doctor. Measures that have been helpful in the past, pre-cancer, could be inappropriate now.

- *American Cancer Society's Guide to Complementary and Alternative Cancer Methods* (American Cancer Society, 2000) is a 400-plus-page book that reviews hundreds of specific treatments, from acupuncture to essiac tea to shamanism. Each therapy is described in detail, with relevant medical citations. Purchase at bookstores or by calling ACS at 888-227-5552.

- The National Center for Complementary and Alternative Medicine (NCCAM) of the National Institutes of Health provides general information on CAM as well as fact sheets about some specific treatments (888-644-6226; *http://nccam.nih.gov*).

- CancerGuide, the web site of respected cancer patient advocate Steve Dunn, offers a thoughtful, balanced approach to CAM. His essay on evaluating unconventional therapies is especially helpful: *http://www. cancerguide.org/alternative.html*.

- The Alternative Medicine section of Health Care Information Resources (*http://www-hsl.mcmaster.ca/tomflem/altmed.html*) provides a comprehensive annotated list of links to online information about alternative medicine. The list is maintained by Tom Flemming, head of public services at the McMaster University Health Sciences Library in Ontario, Canada.

- *The People's Pharmacy: Guide to Home and Herbal Remedies*, by Joe Graedon and Teresa Graedon (Griffin Trade Paperback, 2001), offers extensive information about popular treatments for common problems, including ailments that cancer patients may experience, such as nausea and depression.

- The Office of Dietary Supplements of the National Institutes of Health provides scientific and popular information about nutritional supplements. While it can't respond to individual questions, it offers information sheets and publications, both in print and on its web site (301-435-2920; *http://dietary-supplements.info.nih.gov*).

- The Food and Nutrition Information Center of the U.S. Department of Agriculture offers information about diet and nutrition, including vitamins, minerals, supplements, and herbal products (301-504-5719; *http://www.nal.usda.gov/fnic*).

- Commonweal, a California-based health organization sympathetic to CAM, offers extensive information for cancer patients on its web site (*http://www.commonweal.org/canproj.html*), including the full text of a 1994 book by Michael Lerner, president and founder of Commonweal, titled *Choices in Healing: Integrating the Best of Conventional and Complementary Approaches to Cancer.*

- Quackwatch (*http://www.quackwatch.com*) is a nonprofit corporation whose purpose is to combat health-related fraud and fallacies. Its web site contains comprehensive, detailed—and highly skeptical—information about many specific CAM treatments.

Talking to Your Doctor about CAM

To give you the best care, your doctor needs to know about all the therapies you are using. Unfortunately, many patients are reluctant to discuss CAM with their doctors. If you feel this way, ask yourself why. Here are some common issues—and solutions:

- Are you worried that the doctor will criticize you for using a nonstandard treatment? Perhaps you'd find it easier to talk to your oncology nurse first. Nurses often take more time for discussion, and may have more information about CAM therapies.

- Is your reluctance part of a larger problem of communication with this particular physician? If so, you might want to consider finding another doctor with whom you feel more comfortable.

- Are you embarrassed about this particular treatment? In that case, perhaps you need to learn more about it so that you can decide if you're comfortable using it or would rather stop.

Reading with a Critical Eye

As you explore CAM treatments, you may read persuasive articles by practitioners and thrilling testimonials from other cancer survivors. Below are questions to ask yourself if you encounter claims that a nonstandard treatment can cure cancer.

- What evidence is there that the patients really had cancer? What type and stage of cancer was it? How was this confirmed?

- What conventional therapies did they receive—and might these treatments account for some or all of the success?

- Was the treatment compared to anything else, such as a placebo or a standard therapy?

- How many people who have received the therapy were *not* helped?

- How was it determined that patients were cured?

- How long after the treatment were they followed to be sure the cancer didn't return?

If Your Doctor Says No

When you're convinced that a complementary treatment would help you, it's upsetting and puzzling if your doctor disagrees. Perhaps it's just prejudice or lack of information, or maybe there's an important reason to advise against it. Here are some suggestions for dealing with the situation:

- Give your doctor printed information with evidence in favor of this treatment, such as material from the *American Cancer Society's Guide to Complementary and Alternative Cancer Methods*, mentioned earlier.

- Ask the doctor to explain the negative recommendation. Sometimes it's helpful to have a trusted friend or relative accompany you both for support and to help you understand and evaluate what your doctor is saying.

- Ask about other options that might be able to accomplish what you're hoping to achieve with the method you're asking about.

- If you're still uncertain about what to do, get a second opinion from another trusted physician who is more open-minded about CAM.

How to Select a CAM Practitioner

Reread the advice in Chapter 10 about finding a doctor. The issues are similar when you're seeking referrals and evaluating a CAM caregiver. Here are additional suggestions:

Where to Get Reliable Referrals

Start by talking to your doctor or oncology nurse. Find out what services are available where you're being treated. Other patients and support groups may have suggestions.

Does Insurance Cover CAM Treatment?

Because so many patients use complementary and alternative therapies, some insurers and HMOs pay for them. However, the coverage may be more limited than it is for conventional medicine. Insurers
are most likely to cover measures for which there is accepted scientific
evidence of effectiveness. Two suggestions:

- Before you start treatment, discuss insurance concerns with your
conventional healthcare provider and your insurance company
or HMO. Ask the CAM practitioner for recommendations on
getting coverage. Sometimes other patients can offer advice on
dealing with insurance companies.

- Keep records of your payments for CAM treatments if your
insurer refuses to cover them. You may be able to appeal this
decision. But even if you can't, the expenses *may* be tax-
deductible. See the current edition of Internal Revenue Service
Publication 502, *Medical and Dental Expenses*, for the latest
information on what is and is not tax deductible as a medical
expense. The publication is available at the IRS web site
(*http://www.irs.gov*) or from your local IRS office, which is listed
in the white pages of your telephone directory.

As you research the treatment, you'll learn about its leading organizations, schools, and practitioners. Call any of these and ask for a referral to
someone in your area. As with M.D.s, it's best to talk to several practitioners
before you select one, since they don't all work in the same way.

Questions to Ask

Here are questions to ask a CAM practitioner at your first meeting:

- What training and experience and certification do you have?

- Are you licensed to practice in your field?

- Are you willing to work with my oncologist or primary care physician?

- What does treatment consist of?

- How does it work? What is the evidence of its effectiveness and safety?

- What benefits can I expect? When should I expect to see these effects? How long will they last?

- What is the goal of treatment—to relieve symptoms or side effects, or to improve the efficacy of standard medical treatment? Note: if the practitioner claims to be able to cure your disease, consider that a serious warning sign. See box below for other red flags.

Red Flags

- A warning that you can't trust your doctor or that conventional medicine is suppressing information about an effective cancer treatment

- A recommendation that you stop conventional therapies

- Terms like "miracle," "breakthrough," "cure," or "new discovery"

- Secret ingredients or methods

- Claims based only on testimonials and anecdotes

- A promise that the treatment can cure all cancers

- A method promoted only in the popular media—on television, in magazines—and not discussed in scientific journals

- An office that seems unclean or unsafe—for instance, sterilization technique seems lax or needles are reused

- An effort to recruit you as a salesperson or to sell you a distributorship

- Attempts to blame you if treatment isn't effective (examples: "I could have cured you if you'd only started sooner" or "You didn't really want to get better")

- What are the possible risks? Can the therapy interfere with conventional measures? If so, in what ways?

- How much will treatment cost? Will my insurance cover it? If so, who handles the billing?

CAM treatments are widely used by cancer patients. Indeed, therapies that today are considered complementary and alternative have been used for centuries in many cultures. We're delighted to see the medical and scientific community acknowledge the significance of CAM and begin to give it the attention and careful scrutiny it deserves.

Without a doubt, some CAM practices are of enormous benefit; others may be less useful or even harmful. As we learn more about these treatments, the most helpful ones will be incorporated into standard medical practice. But even today, people with lung cancer can improve the quality of their lives by judicious use of complementary medicine.

PART VI

Living with Lung Cancer

CHAPTER 16

Treatment Is Finished— Now What?

You think that the further away from surgery, the better off you'll be.
But you have to deal with the fact that it's never over. I don't know if
I'll live another year or ten years or thirty years. But I refuse to let
this stop me from doing the things I want to do.
—Estrea

S aying goodbye to cancer treatment is like leaving home for the first time. You've waited so eagerly for this moment, but when it arrives you may be surprised by mixed feelings. Yes, there's the expected relief and joy. But you may also experience heightened anxiety and sense of loss. Your medical team has been a source of security. However difficult treatment has been, at least you were doing something. Now you wonder: What happens next? Will the cancer come back? How can I stay healthy?

Probably you still have some recovery to do. After surgery, you may need weeks or even months to feel like yourself again. If you've had chemotherapy or radiation, fatigue and other side effects may linger. Over time, some of these symptoms should improve and your energy should increase. But finishing treatment for lung cancer is not like getting over the flu. Loss of lung tissue may permanently alter your pulmonary functioning. And you will be a cancer survivor for the rest of your life. This chapter will help you make the transition.

Where Do You Stand Now?

At the end of treatment, you'll be examined and evaluated. Here's what your doctor might say and what it means:

"You're Cured"

If you had surgery for early-stage disease, your surgeon may tell you, "You're cured." That's very good news. It means that no cancer was detected in the tissue margins (healthy lung tissue around the tumor) or in your lymph nodes. However, as we'll explain below, you still need frequent checkups to make sure the disease is discovered early if it returns. Also, we strongly recommend that you speak with a medical oncologist (chemotherapy specialist) and a radiation oncologist to learn if you might benefit from additional treatment. If so, it should begin promptly—adjuvant (postsurgical) treatment is started soon after surgery.

"You're in Complete Remission"

Most oncologists (unlike surgeons) don't use the word "cured," but instead say, "You're in complete remission." This is also very good news. No evidence of the disease can be detected in your body after chemotherapy, radiation, or both. Though you'll need frequent checkups, you now appear to be cancer-free.

"You're in Partial Remission"

Your tumors responded to treatment; they shrank and stopped growing. However, they did not disappear completely and must be monitored carefully. This is a good time to reassess your treatment plan. Consultations with other specialists may be helpful. For example, if your tumor was considered inoperable before treatment but it shrank considerably after chemotherapy, a surgeon could determine if you're now a candidate for surgery.

"The Cancer Is Unchanged"

If your tumor had been growing rapidly and its growth was stopped by radiation or chemotherapy, that's a positive development. At this point, your

What Five-Year Survival Means

I was diagnosed more than seven years ago. People think that after five years, you're cancer-free. But my tumors never disappeared, so I've never been able to start counting. In a day, my life could change again.
　　—Donna P.

Scientists use five-year survival as a research tool; it's a simple measure that allows them to compare the outcomes of different treatments. But five-year survival has no special medical significance. It doesn't even mean that you're in remission. Still, the fifth anniversary of a cancer diagnosis is a very encouraging landmark, one that deserves celebration. And the longer you survive with no active cancer, the better your chances of remaining in remission or cancer-free.

doctors may suggest another approach. For instance, if you've had chemotherapy, you might try a different drug; or radiation may be recommended. Lung cancer treatment is advancing rapidly, so consultations with leading specialists could be valuable.

In the beginning, my family and friends thought I was going to die tomorrow. They'd tell each other, "We'd better go see Glenn because he's not going to be around for much longer." Now they think, "He's not dead yet, so he must be cured." They don't have a clue about what's happening with me.
　　—Glenn

"Your Tumors Are Still Growing"

If you've endured difficult treatment, it's terribly disappointing to learn that it didn't work. But we want to emphasize that there are almost always

> When cancer advances despite chemotherapy,
> doctors sometimes tell the patient:
> *You failed treatment.*
> We think it's much more appropriate to say:
> *The treatment failed you.*

more options. If your doctors aren't sure what to try next, get a second opinion. Your best bet could be a clinical trial (see Chapter 14).

"You Have Metastatic Sites"

During treatment, your doctors may learn that the disease has spread beyond your lungs. This is devastating news—especially if you were told initially that the cancer was found early. Get second opinions from a surgeon, a medical oncologist, and a radiation oncologist; ask about clinical trials. There's still hope that treatment could give you months or years of high-quality time, even if a cure is very unlikely.

———

It's like diabetes. I'm not dying from my lung cancer, but it can't be cured. When it's acting up you treat it; when it isn't, you don't.
—Donna M.

———

Follow-up Care for
Lung Cancer Survivors

Estrea was surprised when her doctors suggested no further monitoring after her successful surgery:

I was very lucky. They couldn't see any other cancerous tissue in the lobe that was removed; it wasn't in my lymph nodes; there were no metastases. The doctor said, "We got it all and as far as I'm

*concerned, you're cured." But I knew there was a thing called
recurrence and "as far as I'm concerned" meant there was a reason
for skepticism.*

Unfortunately, some doctors don't realize that lung cancer survivors
always need follow-up care, even if they've been pronounced "cured" or "in
complete remission." Regular checkups and tests are vitally important,
because anyone who has had this disease is at significantly higher risk for a
recurrent cancer (reemergence of the original cancer) or a ***new primary*** (a
new, unrelated tumor):

- Invisible traces of the cancer may remain after treatment.

- Whatever caused this lung cancer—whether it was smoking, exposure to
  other lung carcinogens, or genetic vulnerability—might cause another.

- Radiation therapy and certain kinds of chemotherapy increase the risk
  of subsequent cancer, though this problem has been minimized by
  advances in treatment techniques.

What Is the Goal of Treatment?

Treatment goals vary. Sometimes the aim is to cure. But when lung
cancer is advanced, a cure may be very unlikely. In that case, treatment attempts to prolong life or to maintain the best possible quality
of life; this approach is called ***palliative care*** or ***comfort care.***

Radiation and chemotherapy are used for palliation as well as for
curative treatment. They can shrink tumors to reduce symptoms like
pain, breathlessness, or coughing. Palliative treatments can allow
patients to live more comfortably for extra weeks, months, or even
years. Because the goal is to improve quality of life rather than to cure,
treatment may be modified for comfort and convenience. For example, chemotherapy doses may be lower to prevent side effects.

Doctors and patients don't always discuss treatment goals clearly.
Some patients don't understand the distinction between curative and
palliative treatment. As a result, they may be taken by surprise when
their tumors begin to grow again after therapy they assumed would
cure them.

We recommend that all lung cancer survivors be followed by an oncologist or pulmonologist (chest doctor) who specializes in the disease and keeps abreast of the latest advances in lung cancer detection. Spiral CT and PET have already become important tools. In development are other imaging procedures, sensitive tests of blood and sputum, and other new ways to find any recurrence of lung cancer at earlier stages than ever before. If you prefer to be followed by your primary care doctor—or if your insurance company will not cover routine checkups with a specialist—ask your doctor to speak with an oncologist about your case. Stay informed yourself by joining a lung cancer support group or an advocacy organization like ALCASE.

How Frequently Should You Be Checked?

This is a question to discuss with your doctor, who is familiar with your particular situation—including not only your medical condition but also any constraints placed upon you by insurance, location, and financial resources. Also to be considered are your feelings about follow-up visits. Some lung cancer survivors are eager to be followed closely; they request frequent appointments and are willing to pay for medical visits that insurance doesn't cover. Others can't afford to do this. Or they find checkups so anxiety-provoking that less frequent visits are desirable.

For lung cancer survivors with advanced disease—those who are not cured or in complete remission, and whose remaining tumors are inoperable—most oncologists and insurers follow the guidelines of the American Society of Clinical Oncology (ASCO), quoted on the next page.

Unfortunately, we don't yet have similar guidelines for people whose disease was found early and apparently cured. However, we do know that they are at high risk and need careful monitoring. Therefore we suggest that they too follow the ASCO recommendations, unless their doctor advises more frequent appointments. And we strongly recommend that all lung cancer survivors have a CT scan at least annually.

If you experience changes that suggest a problem,
call your doctor immediately. Don't wait for a scheduled checkup.

What Tests Should You Have?

The following advice may be revised as technology and our knowledge progress. But based on current information, as well as the ASCO guidelines, we recommend that every lung cancer survivor have the following examinations and tests at each checkup:

A Complete Physical Examination

The examination should include blood counts and a pulmonary function test, as well as a manual check for enlarged lymph nodes. The doctor should look for any evidence of lung cancer or metastases, as well as for other health problems for which lung cancer survivors are at risk:

- Medical conditions—such as heart disease, blood clots in the legs, emphysema, and chronic bronchitis—caused by smoking and other factors responsible for the cancer

- Other smoking-related cancers, including bladder, kidney, and head and neck cancer.

- Long-term side effects of chemotherapy and radiation, such as neuropathy or pulmonary fibrosis, as well as infections or cancers that can result from immune system damage

---

Follow-up Recommendations from the American Society of Clinical Oncology

You will need to continue to have medical checkups after your treatment has ended. If the goal of your treatment is to extend your life and you have no symptoms, your doctor should examine you every three months for two years, then every six months for three years, then once a year.

It may be recommended that you have a CT scan, an MRI test, or a PET scan done after treatment ends. Your doctor can compare the results of this test with tests done earlier and with tests that will be done during your medical checkups in order to evaluate your condition. Chest x-rays and other tests, such as bronchoscopy, complete blood cell count, and other routine tests, may be done as part of these follow-up examinations, depending on the symptoms you may be having. Extensive testing is not done on a routine basis for patients who have no symptoms.

From *A Patient's Guide: Advanced Lung Cancer Treatment.* Copyright 2001 by the American Society of Clinical Oncology (ASCO). Reprinted with permission.

Spiral CT Scan

If you're in complete remission, an annual CT will check that your lungs remain cancer free. If tumors are still present after treatment, the scans look for growth and may need to be done more frequently. Best for this purpose are three-dimensional images, which can reveal growth that is invisible when only two dimensions are shown. Ask your radiology team if they're using this technology. We recommend against relying on chest x-rays for these important checkups, since spiral CT is far more sensitive. This recommendation might change in the future as techniques for early diagnosis of lung cancer advance.

Talking to Your Doctor

Don't be surprised if you find follow-up medical visits very stressful. Try to make them reassuring too. When your doctor asks, "How are you?" don't reply with an automatic "Fine." Discuss any lingering symptoms. Write down your concerns ahead of time or bring a close friend or relative who will speak up if you leave something out.

Ask your doctor for referrals if you think that specialized assistance would facilitate your return to normal life:

- **Pulmonary rehabilitation therapist** if you're suffering from breathlessness, fatigue, or lack of energy

- **Physical therapist** if you're experiencing muscle aches and stiffness, or if you want a safe plan for becoming more active

- **Nutritionist** if you've lost too much weight during treatment and are still having trouble eating, or if you want to improve your diet

- **Acupuncturist** if you're experiencing lingering pain from surgery

- **Counselor,** such as a psychologist or social worker, if you need help with difficult emotions or problems in your relationships

- **Support groups** for you and for your family if you feel you would benefit from participation

———

The fear of recurrence is intense and horrible. But you have to ignore it to live. There are times when you can ignore it very easily. Then

there are times when you allow yourself to fall into that pit. If I get a headache, I think, "Oh my God—I have to schedule an MRI." I'm so afraid that something is wrong. Then it will turn out I've been drinking too much coffee.
    —Glenn

Reducing the Risk That Cancer Will Return

It's never too late to make healthy lifestyle changes! Take advantage of the strong motivation you feel now. Old habits often lose their grip during treatment. The more you do to stay healthy, the more in control and the better you will feel.

Consider Clinical Trials Aimed at Prevention

If you're in complete remission, look for chemoprevention trials—studies of nontoxic agents that may prevent lung cancer. If you're in partial remission, look for trials designed to prevent tumor growth. See Chapter 14 for information about clinical trials.

Minimize Your Exposure to Carcinogens

Review your risk factors (see Chapter 6) to see what can be changed. Do everything in your power to quit smoking if you haven't already (see Chapter 7).

Resume (or Begin) Regular Exercise

When you're recovering from treatment, merely thinking about exercise can be exhausting. However, if you make a conservative start and advance slowly but consistently, you will progress.

Physical activity reduces lung cancer risk and improves lung health generally. As your lungs recover, you'll feel stronger and more energetic; lingering fatigue will ease. Exercise also has proven benefits for mood: it's as

Exercise Cautions for Lung Cancer Survivors

I f you were active before your diagnosis, you will need to modify your previous level of exercise, at least at first. If you've been sedentary, you should start at a safe level. Slowly increase the duration and intensity of exercise, giving your body a chance to adjust.

Always discuss exercise plans with your doctor and report any specific symptoms or concerns.

Problem	Cautions
Fatigue, muscle weakness, or breathlessness	Adjust duration and intensity of exercise to match capacity. Increase cautiously as symptoms improve.
Peripheral neuropathy (loss of sensation in legs and arms)	Be careful about activities that require balance and coordination.
Leukopenia (insufficient white blood cells)	Avoid activities that might lead to infections or injuries, such as contact sports or swimming in a pool.
Anemia (insufficient red blood cells)	Limit exercise intensity to prevent fatigue.
Thrombocytopenia (insufficient platelets)	Avoid activities that might lead to injuries and bleeding, such as contact or risky sports.
Bone metastases	Avoid activities that might cause fractures, such as high-impact aerobic exercise or contact sports.

Adapted with the permission of Kerry S. Courneya, Ph.D., from "Coping with Cancer—Can Exercise Help?" by K. S. Courneya, J. R. Mackey, and L. W. Jones, in *The Physician and Sportsmedicine*, May 2000, Vol. 28:5.

effective as medication for mild depression and anxiety, but without the potential side effects of drugs. Convinced? See page 179 for an overview of appropriate exercises.

Eat Well

A nutritious diet—one that's low in fat and includes plenty of fruits and vegetables—reduces lung cancer risk. Good food also fuels your recovery by supporting your energy and strength. Nutritional supplements may be helpful, but check with your doctor to make sure there are no contraindications.

Unfortunately, the lingering effects of lung cancer and treatment can interfere with appetite. For example, some painkillers can cause constipation, which can leave you feeling too bloated to eat. If you can't eat properly, talk to your doctor so the cause can be tracked down and resolved. See pages 199–203 for more information on eating problems. Sometimes it's difficult to translate nutrition guidelines into practical menus that you and your family will enjoy. If you need one-on-one help, ask your doctor to refer you to a nutritionist.

▬

I had terrible gastrointestinal problems—pain in my stomach, alternating constipation and diarrhea, difficulty swallowing. It took so much energy to cook. Then when I did, I couldn't eat it anyway. I kept losing weight. People urged me to eat and to have a positive attitude. That upset me so much. Didn't they understand that I know I have to eat? Normally I enjoy food. If I can eat, I do.

My oncologist said, "It's because you're depressed." When you don't know the answer, it's easy to blame depression. I felt I wasn't listened to. Finally a gastroenterologist diagnosed a hernia and an esophageal ulcer.

—Joyce

▬

Taking Stock of Your Life and Yourself

During treatment you longed to resume your normal life. Now that treatment is over, you may be surprised to find that "normal" means something new. For most people, lung cancer is a transforming experience. They see themselves, their family, and their friends differently. Life will go on, but it won't be the same.

Finding New Pleasure in Life

The ordinary becomes precious after illness threatens to snatch it away. Many lung cancer survivors feel altered by their new outlook. Here's how Glenn describes it:

> A year before I was diagnosed, we bought a dream home in the hills overlooking a bay. You can sit on our deck and see three bridges. On July Fourth, you can see fireworks in four different cities. Before my diagnosis, I'd be on the deck and I wouldn't look at the view. I could only see the green metal railing that either I'd have to paint (which I didn't want to do) or I'd have to pay someone else to paint. Now I see the view, not the railing. That's how my life has changed.

Different Priorities

A close encounter with a life-threatening illness is a potent reminder of what's important and what's not. Survivors say that lung cancer rearranges their priorities. This often means letting go of the trivial and focusing on the substantive and enriching aspects of your life.

———

> I'm living each day as if it were my last. I thought I did that before my diagnosis, but I didn't. My husband and I had wanted to go on trips but I wouldn't take time from work. Since my diagnosis we've gone to Hawaii a couple of times; we went to New York and had a great time there. I've seen couples who say they'll travel when they retire. Then one of them gets cancer and dies. I've learned that you do it now.
> —Donna M.

———

With new priorities come new goals and activities. It's not uncommon for lung cancer survivors to make major changes in their lives. Estrea says:

Before cancer and after cancer, I'm a very different person. Everything I do now is affected—from the littlest things like buying a pair of shoes, up to big things like changing career paths. I quit my job and went back to a company that I used to work for and didn't appreciate.

Personal Relationships

Cancer, like other life crises, often reveals the strengths—and weaknesses—of your relationships. You may feel a new closeness to those family and members and friends who reached out to help you. Phil said:

There are perverse benefits. I'm closer to my wife, my children, my friends, because we're dealing with shortened time. Love is extended to you in ways that you never would have expected. A friend walked three miles to see me in the hospital, because his wife had their car. Two sets of friends have assured my wife that she doesn't need to worry about paying for college.

On the other hand, you may have mixed feelings about the friends who drifted away because they couldn't cope with your disease (and who may drift back now that you've finished treatment). Because you've changed, you may feel out of synch with people untouched by cancer.

A woman I know slightly came up to me in church and said, "What's your prognosis these days?" I wanted to say, "Give me a calendar and I'll let you know how many days I have left."
—*Tracy*

Expect a period of readjustment as normal life resumes. You'll probably still feel in need of support—but the people who have been your bulwarks may become less tolerant and more demanding. This is understandable: While you were undergoing treatment, family members, friends, and colleagues shouldered many extra burdens. To protect you, they suppressed their own needs and feelings. Children were on their best behavior. Now that your treatment is over, they may feel—with some justification—that it's their turn to be nurtured. Youngsters may become needy or clingy; they may begin to act out in school or at home, because it now seems safe to do so.

This is a time for clear communication. Express your appreciation for all your family and friends have done. But also help everyone to understand how long it takes to recover from the physical, emotional, and mental toll of lung cancer. A support group can be very beneficial, even if you haven't participated in one before. (See page 137 for suggestions on finding a group.)

If Cancer Returns

An ominous spot appears on the CT scan of a previously clear lung; a quiet tumor begins to grow; troubling symptoms reveal a new metastasis. The cancer, previously beaten into submission, is back. Or an unrelated tumor has emerged. Cancer may reappear shortly after treatment or years later.

Your first cancer diagnosis probably was a surprise. Most likely, you had no idea what to expect. You struggled to learn a new vocabulary; you coped with unfamiliar treatments. The second time around, there's less shock and you're a veteran. But you may feel greater dread because you know what treatment will entail. Also, it's harder to feel optimistic.

Before you're treated, your doctors will check to see if the latest cancer is a recurrence, with the same type of cancer cells as the first, or (less likely) a new primary, an unrelated tumor with a different kind of cells. Treatment depends on the answer. For example, if you've had a recurrence soon after completing chemotherapy, a new drug may be recommended. That's because the cells that are growing could be resistant to the drugs used previously. Experimental therapies could be helpful now. See Chapter 14 for information on locating and participating in clinical trials.

Physicians sometimes hesitate to offer more treatment to people whose cancer has come back. But this should be the patient's decision. If your health can withstand further treatment and you wish to proceed, let your doctor know. If necessary, seek care elsewhere to find a physician who will support your decision. Some long-term lung cancer survivors receive many different treatments over the years.

Ken Giddes was diagnosed with stage I non-small cell lung cancer in 1993. A year later the cancer recurred; this time it was stage IV. His response was to seek treatment—and to reach out to others.

Ken survived nearly eight years after his diagnosis. During that time he helped thousands of cancer patients. With support from his employer,

Republic Financial Corporation, Ken developed the Caring Ambassadors Program, through which he traveled around the country talking with other survivors about living with lung cancer. He served ALCASE not only as vice chair of the board of directors, but as an active Phone Buddy. Ken died January 27, 2001, surrounded by his family. His memory and his words remain an inspiration to all who knew him. We hope they will inspire you too.

> *I live in gratitude and wonder every day, for I know I am what every oncologist who treats people with lung cancer hopes for the patient. I am experiencing long-term survival after being diagnosed with stage IV lung cancer.*
>
> *Like climbing a mountain, becoming a cancer survivor isn't easy. I do it with a lot of luck; excellent treatment; careful monitoring by trained oncology professionals; the love and support of my wife, Barbara, and my other family members and friends; regular exercise; a good diet and nutrients; and my deep faith in God. I have struggled up one slope after another, and am doing my best to guide others who are facing this illness to climb the mountain with me—because no one should have to make the climb alone.*

CHAPTER 17

Optimizing the Quality of Your Life

All the support helped me get better. Parents at my children's school brought meals over when I was having treatment. My brother and sister came from the East Coast to help out any way they could. Neighbors expressed interest and concern. I was on prayer lists. Everyone hugged me. No one knew how long I'd be around. But after a year, I wanted to put all that behind me and to get back to leading a normal life.
—Ben

———

Returning to normal life—not merely staying alive—is the goal of treatment, whether you're in remission or living with active disease. This chapter discusses the most common physical and emotional difficulties that lung cancer survivors face: fatigue, breathlessness, pain, depression and anxiety, and sexual problems. All can interfere with the quality of your life, and all can be addressed.

Fatigue

Lung cancer survivors say that fatigue is the most debilitating problem associated with the disease and its treatment. This isn't ordinary end-of-the-day fatigue; sleep brings no relief. Though fatigue plagues survivors of all kinds of cancer—76 percent of patients reported the problem in a 1999 *Oncology* survey—it's usually worse for those with lung cancer.

Fatigue can interfere with your ability to think, steal your energy, and leave you unable to work or carry out everyday chores. It can rob you of time with your loved ones and everything else that makes life enjoyable. Fatigue may decline over time after treatment ends. If not, you can do something about it.

Why You're So Tired

Fatigue is your body's way of forcing you to slow down when your cells aren't getting enough oxygen. Once you and your doctor figure out the cause of the oxygen deficit, you'll know how to relieve the problem. Here are the most common reasons:

- **Loss of lung tissue:** Your pulmonary system, which brings oxygen into your body and moves carbon dioxide out, is overtaxed. As you recover, your body can compensate somewhat.

- **Anemia (insufficient red blood cells):** As we explained in Chapter 12, anemia can be treated. Unfortunately, it's often neglected. In the 1999 *Oncology* survey mentioned above, a third of the patients had been diagnosed with anemia, but only 9 percent had received treatment. ALCASE frequently hears about patients who are bedridden because of exhaustion and who aren't receiving therapy for anemia even though their red blood cell counts are significantly below normal. Sometimes their doctors tell them, "This is what you can expect if you've had lung cancer." But that's not true! Addressing the anemia can reduce fatigue considerably.

- **Muscle weakness:** Exercise helps fatigue, because physical activity addresses muscle weakness.

- **Depression:** This too is a treatable problem. We'll have more to say about depression later in this chapter.

- **Other physical problems:** Possibilities include emphysema, chronic bronchitis, heart disease, or a developing tumor. That's why it's so important to track down the cause of your fatigue.

What You Can Do

As you recover, your lungs should regain strength; you'll become more active and your muscles will get stronger. Treating anemia or depression will also help. The following healthy lifestyle changes can speed the process:

Tips for Conserving Energy

- Plan your day to take advantage of the times when you usually feel most awake and energetic.

- Relax your housekeeping standards and simplify chores. Wear clothing that doesn't need ironing or other special care; send laundry out to be cleaned; shop online or by telephone.

- Accept offers of help or hire people to assist you. If possible, have a friend coordinate the helpers, since that can be tiring too.

- Minimize the time you spend in bed. Exercise helps strengthen your heart, lungs, and muscles—and lifts depression. See page 179 for suggestions.

- Eat well and pay attention to your fluid intake. Inadequate nutrition and dehydration can contribute to fatigue.

- Minimize stress, which drains energy. Include enjoyable activities in your life—they're therapeutic.

- Be realistic about what you can do. Learn to say no.

———

I retired last February. Making that decision was hard. When I quit, I felt I was giving in to the cancer. But I didn't have the energy to handle my career plus being a mother and wife. Now I can nap in the afternoon and spend time later with my daughter, Jessica. I can go to dinner and a movie with my husband, Jon. I miss my job terribly, but I know I did the right thing.
  —Donna P.

———

For more information about fatigue:

- The National Cancer Institute's PDQ for patients on cancer fatigue is available online (*http://www.cancer.gov*) or by calling 800-4-CANCER.

- The Oncology Nursing Society maintains a web site focused on cancer symptoms, with a special section about fatigue: *http://www.cancer symptoms.org.*

- The Association of Cancer Online Resources (ACOR) hosts online discussion groups for people with cancer, including one about fatigue (*http://listserv.acor.org/archives/cancer-fatigue.html*).

- Cancer Care's web site has a valuable special section on cancer-related fatigue (*http://www.cancercare.org/fatigue*).

Breathlessness

Breathlessness—called *dyspnea* or air hunger—is a common symptom of lung cancer (see pages 101–103). The problem may persist through treatment, or it may appear afterward. If dyspnea is mild, you don't notice shortness of breath unless you exert yourself. When it's severe, you feel breathless even at rest. Tell your doctor if you're experiencing dyspnea so the reason can be tracked down and addressed.

What Causes Dyspnea?

Breathlessness may be related to cancer treatment. As your lungs recover, dyspnea may decrease. But the problem also could signal anemia, heart disease, anxiety, or other pulmonary conditions such as emphysema or asthma. Sometimes the cause is a tumor that's obstructing an airway or secreting fluid into the lungs. When these problems are resolved or improved, dyspnea eases.

What You Can Do

A few simple measures help prevent breathlessness:

- Practice abdominal breathing (see page 28–29) and use an inspiratory muscle trainer (see page 178) to strengthen the muscles used in respiration.

- Start a walking program (see page 74) to rehabilitate your lungs.

- Elevate the head of your bed or use extra pillows if you often become breathless at night.

When You Can't Catch Your Breath

An episode of acute dsypnea is terrifying, but fear exacerbates the problem. Some tricks to try:

• Do controlled breathing. Breathe in through your nose, counting the seconds until your lungs are filled. Exhale through pursed lips, taking twice as many seconds as you did to inhale.

• Use a relaxation technique. See Chapter 15 for examples. Relaxing your arms and shoulders is particularly helpful.

• Increase air movement: open a window or set up a fan to blow cool air against your face.

If dyspnea is severe, ask your doctor about measures to relieve it. Possibilities include medication and supplemental oxygen. Tumors that cause breathlessness can be treated with chemotherapy, radiation (including brachytherapy—see pages 220–221), surgery (including photodynamic therapy—see page 173), and insertion of an airway stent (see box on next page).

For more information see *Shortness of Breath: A Guide to Better Living and Breathing*, by Andrew Ries, M.D., and associates (Mosby, 2000), a book with many suggestions for dealing with chronic dyspnea.

Pain

Cancer doesn't have to hurt. Yet all too often it does. According to statistics from the American Society of Clinical Oncology (ASCO), about 60 to 90 percent of patients with advanced cancer experience pain; of those, a third describe their pain as moderate to severe. This suffering takes a terrible toll on health and on quality of life. If you're in pain, you can't eat or sleep well, and you're vulnerable to depression. That's why adequate pain relief is such an important part of cancer care.

Unfortunately, as the ASCO statistics suggest, there's a distressing gap between state-of-the-art pain management and the inadequate responses by

Airway Stents to Relieve Breathlessness

Breathlessness may be caused by a tumor that's inside an air passage or pressing against it and causing *stenosis* (narrowing or constriction). One way to relieve symptoms quickly is to implant a *stent*—a short tube made of silicone, metal, or a combination—in the affected section to hold the airway open.

Stents are implanted under general anesthesia with the help of a bronchoscope, a viewing instrument. The bronchoscope carries the stent through the nose or mouth and down the airway to the blocked area. Patients usually wake up to find their breathlessness dramatically reduced. Occasionally, stents cause scarring or other complications, or they move out of position and the airway closes again. If there's a problem, the procedure usually can be repeated.

doctors who don't follow current approaches. During checkups, your doctor should question you about pain. If not, raise the issue yourself. Don't minimize the amount of pain you feel, and never hesitate to advocate persistently for yourself if you're suffering from pain.

What Causes Cancer Pain?

Lung cancer or its treatment can cause pain in several ways:

- Surgery can leave painful scars because nerves were cut.

- A tumor growing inside the lungs may press against the ribs, the spine, or nerves that lead to the arms or back.

- Lung metastases to the brain can cause headaches because the tumor is pressing against nerves or against the skull.

- Metastases to the bone—which enlarge bones and may cause them to press against nerves—can produce pain in the ribs, breastbone, sternum, leg bones, or spine.

- Chemotherapy can cause neuropathy (see pages 207–208), which makes it painful to use the hands and feet.

Pain or Breathlessness That Requires Immediate Attention

Lung cancer survivors are vulnerable to blood clotting problems, which can cause heart attack, stroke, or *pulmonary embolism* (a clot that blocks major vessels in the lungs). Notify your doctor immediately if you experience any of the following:

• Unaccustomed breathlessness, especially if it appears suddenly

• An unusually severe headache

• Pain in your chest that lasts for more than five minutes

• Unexplained sudden pain in your left arm or shoulder

If you take blood thinners, such as heparin (Lovenox) or warfarin (Coumadin), maintain a consistent intake of vitamin K, which can affect the action of your medication. Talk to your doctor before taking herbs or supplements or making dietary changes.

• Radiation can produce painful tissue damage, called fibrosis, which feels like the stiffness and aching of arthritis.

As a lung cancer survivor, you will be alert to pain—and worried about what it might mean. While it's very important to check out anything new and persistent, don't panic! The most likely causes are relatively harmless. If your back hurts, it's probably muscle strain; if your shoulders ache, it's most likely tension or too many hours hunched over a desk.

How to Describe Your Pain

The more precisely you describe your pain, the more easily your doctor can identify the cause and treat it effectively. Keep a pain diary that includes key information:

• **Time:** When you feel pain and for how long.

Pain Intensity Scale

Pain is difficult to measure, because it's purely subjective—no one else can know what your pain feels like to you. Your doctor may ask you to rate your pain on a scale of 0 (no pain) to 10. These guidelines can help.

Score	Description
1 to 2	Pain is mild. It's a tolerable annoyance that isn't noticeable all the time.
3 to 4	Pain is distracting and irritating. It's noticeable most of the time, but doesn't interfere with everyday activities.
5 to 6	Pain is disruptive and stressful. It's always noticeable, but ordinary tasks can be performed with effort.
7 to 8	Pain is intrusive and upsetting. It's difficult to sleep, converse, or carry out everyday tasks.
9 to 10	Pain is agonizing and overwhelming, and may cause loss of consciousness. Ordinary activities are impossible.

- **Circumstances:** Factors that trigger pain, such as particular activities or positions.

- **Location:** Where in your body you feel pain.

- **Sensations:** Nature of the pain. Is it sharp or dull? Deep or superficial? Tingling, aching, pinching, or stabbing?

- **Intensity:** Rate the pain on a scale of 0 to 10, where 0 is absence of pain and 10 is the worst pain imaginable. (See box above.)

Dealing with the Cause

When pain is caused by a tumor, eliminating or at least shrinking it is best. If there's hope of removing all trace of the cancer, surgery might be used. But if cancer is advanced, you and your doctor will weigh the discomfort of surgery against the benefits of pain relief. When the goal is palliation (that is, to improve comfort), these are the measures most commonly used for tumor-caused pain:

- External radiation for tumors in the lungs and airways, or for metastases in bone or the brain, which are difficult to treat with chemotherapy or surgery

- Internal radiation (brachytherapy) to shrink painful tumors in the airways

- Photodynamic therapy for painful airway tumors

- Chemotherapy to shrink pain-causing tumors, even if they can't be eliminated entirely

---

Five Myths That Interfere with Pain Relief

Myth #1: Good patients don't complain.

When you tell your doctor you're in pain, you're not complaining—you're providing the information needed to treat you properly.

Myth #2: Nothing can be done for cancer pain.

Cancer pain can nearly always be relieved. Many different approaches are available. If one doesn't work, another might.

Myth #3: Pain medication is addictive.

People who take narcotic pain medication for treatment of cancer pain rarely become addicted to it. They don't develop the cravings and out-of-control behavior that characterize drug addicts.

Myth #4: Pain medication should be used sparingly and saved for when it's really needed.

On the contrary, pain relief is most effective when given early. Once pain takes hold, more medication is needed to bring it under control.

Myth #5: Pain medication leaves patients doped up and groggy.

Side effects may occur when you begin taking pain medication, but they usually ease after a few days. If not, ask your doctor what can be done.

New Approaches to Pain Management

The underlying cause of pain can't always be addressed. But pain control is always possible. *You do not have to suffer.*

If you're not familiar with the modern arsenal of pain relief measures, you'll be happily surprised by the new approaches and new attitudes. In the past, medication was prescribed PRN (from the Latin *pro re nata*, meaning "as necessary"); in other words, it was given only in response to pain. At that point, pain may be difficult or impossible to control. The current approach is to prescribe medication before pain becomes intense.

Trial and error may be necessary to find the relief measures that work most effectively and with minimal side effects. Keep a pain diary (see instructions above on describing your pain) and discuss your pain with your doctor. Don't hold back information in a misguided effort to seem stoical. Pain is detrimental to your health. If your regular doctor can't help or has antiquated attitudes toward pain control, ask for a referral to a pain management specialist.

Medications

You and your doctor may need to experiment to find the best way to relieve your pain. If the first *analgesic* (painkiller) you try isn't effective or has unpleasant side effects, perhaps a different dose, a different way of administering the drug, or a different medication would work better. Here are the main types of medication used for pain; they're often combined to boost efficacy:

- **Acetaminophen** (Tylenol and other brands), a nonprescription pain reliever, counters pain of low to moderate intensity.

- **Nonsteroidal anti-inflammatory drugs** (NSAIDs) reduce inflammation as well as pain of low to moderate intensity. Examples are aspirin, ibuprofen (Motrin and other brands), and naproxen sodium (Aleve and other brands). Some are available over the counter; stronger doses require a prescription (which may mean that insurance will cover it).

- **Opioids** (narcotics) relieve more severe pain. They are available only by prescription. Examples include morphine, codeine, fentanyl, meperidine (Demerol), and oxycodone (OxyContin). Opioids usually are combined with nonopioid painkillers, allowing the narcotic part of the dose to be smaller. For instance, some prescription painkillers combine oxy-codone with aspirin (Percodan) or with acetaminophen (Percocet).

- **Antidepressants,** drugs normally used to treat depression, are also effective against pain, especially the burning pain of neuropathy. Bupro-pion (Wellbutrin) is often used with lung cancer patients who have recently given up smoking. (The same medication in smaller doses is sold as Zyban and prescribed to reduce cravings after smoking cessa-tion—see pages 88–90)

- **Tranquilizers,** medications used to counter anxiety, may be helpful for pain as well, since muscle tension can exacerbate discomfort.

- **Anticonvulsants,** prescription medications used against seizures, can control pain too, particularly pain from neuropathy.

- **Corticosteroids** may be prescribed for pain caused by inflammation.

Coping with Side Effects

Unfortunately, pain-relieving drugs may cause side effects. Sometimes the problems disappear in a few days as your body gets used to the medica-

Patient-Controlled Analgesia

*P*atient-controlled analgesia* (PCA) allows you to deliver an "injection" of a painkilling drug via a pump attached to your body. When you press a button on the PCA device, a regulated dose is injected into a small tube that's placed under your skin, in a vein, or in the space around your spinal cord. Most patients obtain superior pain relief with PCA compared with standard treatment in which doses are delivered at regular intervals. Surprisingly, they actually need *less* medication. This method is most commonly used for hospitalized patients—for example, to provide pain relief after surgery. However, portable PCA machines are available, so it's sometimes an option for cancer patients who haven't obtained satisfactory relief from simpler measures.

Breakthrough Pain

People who take medication for chronic cancer pain may experience occasional spikes of pain, called *breakthrough pain*. Sometimes these episodes can be managed by relaxation or self-hypnosis techniques. But if the problem is severe, a quick-acting drug can be used as a supplement. Using a second drug this way is called *rescue medication*.

———

Tumors in my right lung are growing into my ribs, which causes a lot of pain. I take Demerol and OxyContin, but the pain gets worse at night when I'm tired and there are fewer distractions. If I took another Demerol, it would be forty-five minutes before the pain eased up. So I use Actiq. It's like a lollypop. I suck on it and twirl it between my teeth and gums. In five minutes the pain is almost completely gone.
—Donna P.

tion. For example, some people experience temporary sleepiness or nausea when they take opioid painkillers.

If side effects persist, work with your doctor to find a solution:

- Adjust the dose or the timing. For instance, if you experience stomach upset when taking a medication that includes aspirin, it might be helpful to take your dose with meals.

- Try the same medication in a different form, such as a patch instead of a pill. (See box on next page.)

- Try a different drug, which may be just as effective against pain without producing the same difficulties.

- Adopt additional measures to deal with side effects. For example, if you suffer from constipation, a common side effect of opioid pain relievers, your doctor might suggest dietary modifications or a laxative.

Other Pain-Relief Measures

The following do-it-yourself techniques may be sufficient to relieve mild, occasional pain. You can also use them to supplement other measures: they can help you deal with breakthrough pain or with pain for which you've taken a painkiller that needs time to take effect.

- **Relaxation techniques.** Since muscle tension exacerbates pain, relaxation techniques can relieve discomfort (see Chapter 15).

- **Distraction.** As you've probably noticed, you're less bothered by pain when your mind is engaged with something else.

- **Substitute sensations.** Stimulating the skin with nonpainful sensations—heat, cold, pressure, or vibration—sometimes relieves pain. Experiment with hot and cold packs and massage, taking care not to irritate sensitive skin.

Here are three possibilities for pain that resists other treatment:

- **Acupuncture,** which is effective against incision pain, may be helpful. See pages 259–260 for more information.

- **Transcutaneous Electric Nerve Stimulation** (TENS) uses a device to apply mild electric currents to the skin, producing a tingling, buzzing feeling. TENS may block pain signals from nerves to the brain, or it might trigger the release of endorphins, chemicals that act as the body's

---

Same Drug, Different Form

Your doctors can improve your comfort not only by selecting the most appropriate medication, but also by administering the drug in the best way. Pills or capsules sometimes can be given in long-acting form, so that you get continuous relief without having to take medication as often. If it's difficult for you to swallow pills, or if they cause nausea or digestive problems, you may be able to receive the painkiller another way, such as via a skin patch or a rectal suppository.

Pain Relief Problems and Solutions

"My pain medicine doesn't work and my doctor says there's nothing more she can do."

There is nearly always a way to relieve pain from cancer. Ask your doctor to refer you to a pain specialist. Or contact the nearest cancer treatment center. See pages 148–149 for information on finding cancer centers.

"My insurance doesn't cover medication, and I can't afford the pain drug my doctor prescribed."

Most drug companies have programs that provide medication free to those in need (see page 334). In the meantime, your doctor may be able to provide free samples or to suggest a less expensive alternative.

"My doctor prescribed a narcotic for my pain—but my pharmacy doesn't stock it."

Ask your doctor to suggest another place for you to obtain the medication.

own pain relievers. Battery-operated TENS machines can be purchased for home use with a doctor's prescription for as little as $100.

- **Nerve blocks** use local anesthetics or surgery to cut off sensation.

If pain is an ongoing problem, consult these resources, which provide additional information on pain relief:

- *Pain Control: A Guide for People with Cancer and Their Families,* a free 59-page booklet produced by the National Cancer Institute and the American Cancer Society, provides an excellent overview of options. Order from NCI's Cancer Information Service (800-4-CANCER) or the American Cancer Society (800-ACS-2345).

- Cancer-pain.org (*http://www.cancer-pain.org*), a web site from the Association of Cancer Online Resources (ACOR), offers extensive patient-oriented information about pain. ACOR also has an online support group for people with cancer pain (*http://listserv.acor.org/archives/ cancer-pain.html*) as well as a group for people with neuropathy (*http://listserv.acor.org/archives/cancer-neuropathy.html*).

- *Cancer Pain Treatment Guidelines for Patients* is a free booklet published by the National Comprehensive Cancer Network, a consortium of nineteen leading cancer centers, and the American Cancer Society (888-909-NCNN; *http://www.nccn.org*).

- Cancer Care's web site has a comprehensive special section on cancer pain (*http://www.cancercare.org/pain*).

- For annotated links to other pain information online, see Lung Cancer Online (*http://www.lungcanceronline.org/effects/pain.html*).

Depression and Anxiety

One deadly part is the depression. You lose that will to fight; you get a couldn't-care-less attitude about survival and you give up. I went through this. Fortunately, my doctors treated it with antidepressants.
    —*Doug*

Anyone diagnosed with a life-threatening illness experiences powerful negative emotions. Sadness and fear, as well as difficulty sleeping, eating, and concentrating, all come with the territory. In Chapter 9 we discussed immediate emotional responses to a lung cancer diagnosis and offered coping suggestions. Usually the strongest reactions subside with time. But it's normal for painful feelings, most commonly depression coupled with anxiety, to linger even after successful treatment.

A pity party is when you're feeling sorry for yourself—and enjoying it. Sometimes when I'm talking to my sister she'll say, "Are you having a pity party? If you are, I'm not coming."
    —*Tracy*

Signs That Treatment Is Needed

You may be able to cope with mild depression and anxiety by talking to loved ones or by distracting yourself. But if the feelings persist and become disruptive, professional help can make a difference.

Signs to look for:

- Fears or negative feelings—including unhappiness, worthlessness, guilt, and hopelessness—that remain intense rather than gradually improving

- Inability (or unwillingness) to follow medical instructions because of negative emotions

- Loss of pleasure in life or inability to concentrate on activities that previously were important, including work and family events

- Significant disruption of normal eating and sleeping habits, whether too much or too little food or rest

- Preoccupation with death or suicide

Evaluation and Treatment

Physical problems may be at the root of emotional distress. For example, fatigue can cause depression; breathlessness triggers anxiety. Medication may have adverse emotional side effects. A medical evaluation can sort out the causes and determine appropriate treatment.

Depression and anxiety are treated with counseling, medication, or a combination of the two. Anti-anxiety drugs take effect quickly, but antidepressants don't begin to work for three to six weeks. Sometimes it's necessary to try a different drug or to adjust the dose to get relief.

▬▬

My family feels my temper is too short, and I think they're right. They had me first on Paxil, but it didn't help. I took myself off it. Now I'm on Zoloft, which seems to be working. The problem with the drugs is that though they control anxiety, which helps you be more sociable and understanding, they destroy your energy and your sex life.

—Doug

▬▬

Alternative Treatments for Depression and Anxiety

Research suggests that exercise is just as helpful as—and acts more quickly than—medication for mild depression and anxiety. Also useful, especially for anxiety, are the mind-body techniques described in Chapter 15.

Some studies find that St. John's wort, a popular herbal remedy, is effective for mild to moderate depression and typically causes fewer side effects than standard antidepressants. Preliminary research also indicates that S-adenosylmethionine, known as SAM-e, may relieve depression. If you're interested in trying these or any other alternative remedies for depression, talk to your doctor first. Herbs and supplements can interfere with other medications and may cause side effects.

Here are resources for more information about depression and anxiety:

- The National Cancer Institute has free and informative PDQs (Physician Data Queries) for depression and anxiety, covering both diagnosis and treatment (800-4-CANCER; *http://www.cancer.gov/cancerinfo/coping*).

- The Association of Cancer Online Resources (ACOR) hosts an online discussion group about depression for people with cancer (*http://listserv .acor.org/archives/cancer-depression.html*).

Sexual Problems

Sexually, life wasn't the same for me for a long, long time after surgery. I walked around for many months protecting the right side of my body. I wouldn't hug, wouldn't touch. My husband and I had

*individual and couple therapy, which was helpful. But it takes time
to come through the pain and fear.*
　　　—Selma

——

Sexual problems are common among cancer patients, though they're
not often talked about or studied. The difficulties may be compounded by
age-related changes in sexuality, by other illnesses, or by medications used to
treat the cancer or its symptoms.

How Cancer Treatment May Affect Sexuality

Sex may be far from your mind when you're caught up in the crisis of a
lung cancer diagnosis and coping with treatment. But as you recover and
resume normal life, you might become aware of sexual problems. Sometimes
the difficulties are temporary. But don't ignore them if they persist. Anything
that interferes significantly with the quality of your life should be addressed.

Here are some sexual problems that cancer survivors experience:

- Lack of desire. This could be related to depression or fatigue, or to the
  distraction of dealing with a life-threatening illness.

- Fears. You may feel more vulnerable after surgery; you may be concerned about scars from surgery and how your body will look; you
  might worry about being unable to breathe.

- Inadequate lubrication in women, which makes sexual intercourse
  painful.

- Erectile problems in men.

- Changes in orgasm, including weaker sensations, or inability to reach
  orgasm.

What to Do

As underlying physical difficulties improve, sexuality may return to normal. Meanwhile, you can continue to enjoy intimate physical contact despite
sexual problems, even if it's not the same as it was before. Explore the sexual
enhancers that many healthy couples use, such as vibrators (which provide

intense stimulation) and lubricants like Astroglide or Probe (which increase sensitivity and compensate for delayed or reduced lubrication).

Talk to your doctor if you're experiencing sexual problems. If you'd rather see a specialist, ask for a referral to a sex therapist (or see resources below). New medical approaches—Viagra is the best-known example—can address sexual difficulties. Here are sources of information and referrals:

- The American Cancer Society offers two free brochures, each with more than 50 pages of detailed information and practical advice: *Sexuality and Cancer: For the Woman Who Has Cancer and Her Partner* and *Sexuality and Cancer: For the Man Who Has Cancer and His Partner*. Both are available online (*http://www.cancer.org*) or by calling 800-ACS-2345.

- The Association of Cancer Online Resources (ACOR) has online discussion groups for people with cancer about sexual problems and about fertility problems (*http://listserv.acor.org/archives/cancer-sexuality.html* and *http://listserv.acor.org/archives/cancer-fertitily.html*).

- Two reliable companies that sell sexual enhancers are Good Vibrations, whose free catalog is available online (*http://www.goodvibes.com*) or by calling 800-289-8423, and the Xandria Collection, whose web site offers a catalog and extensive information (*http://www.xandria.com*). The Xandria Collection's print catalogs can be ordered by calling 800-242-2823; the cost of the catalogs ($2 to $4) will be deducted from the first order.

- Referrals to a certified sex therapist can be obtained from the American Association of Sex Educators, Counselors and Therapists (804-644-3288; *http://www.aasect.org*).

Additional Resources

In addition to the resources listed above, which deal with specific problems, the following provide useful general information for cancer survivors:

- The National Cancer Institute has an excellent free booklet called *Facing Forward: A Guide for Cancer Survivors*, which covers health, emotions, and practical matters. It's available online (*http://www.cancer.gov/cancerinfo/life-after-treatment*) or by calling 800-4-CANCER.

- The National Coalition for Cancer Survivorship's book *A Cancer Survivor's Almanac: Charting Your Journey*, edited by Barbara Hoffman, addresses medical, emotional, and legal concerns. It's available in bookstores and can be ordered from the organization's web site (*http://www.canceradvocacy.org*) or by calling 877-NCCS-YES.

- The Association of Cancer Online Resources (ACOR) hosts dozens of online discussion groups on cancer, including many specific topics relevant to lung cancer survivors (*http://listserv.acor.org/archives*).

- Lung Cancer Survivors for Change (*http://www.lungcancersurvivors .org*) provides information and an online discussion forum for people who have been treated for lung cancer.

- Lung Cancer Online has links to many online resources that address problems of lung cancer survivors (*http://www.lungcanceronline.org/ effects/index.html*).

Life after lung cancer is never exactly the same as life before. Even with first-rate medical care and a healthy lifestyle, you may have to live with symptoms that you didn't have to live with previously: aches and pains, extra fatigue, and breathlessness. But with good medical support, you can do a lot to minimize these problems.

Among leading cancer experts, quality of life has become an increasing focus. Unfortunately, physicians don't always offer treatment that could bring relief. We urge you to advocate for yourself if necessary. Many cancer patients have discovered that the disease is a continuing lesson in assertiveness training—and their lives are better for it.

CHAPTER 18

A Message for Caregivers

by Peggy McCarthy

Doug was driving a truck as an independent contractor. He was trying to hide his headaches from me, but I knew something was wrong. He was chewing aspirins. He'd come home with white rings around his mouth.

One day I was at a friend's house when my daughter called. Doug had collapsed on the porch. When my friend and I got there, he was sitting at the dining-room table wondering where he was and why we were all looking at him.

Doug is one of those macho men who never had a doctor. We went to my doctor the next day. He did some tests and we left. Later he called and said he had to see Doug right away. We walked into the office thinking we'd get some medication to fix the headaches. The doctor showed us a picture of the brain and said, "This is where your tumor is." I'm waiting for a pill, and it's a brain tumor. Then they did an x-ray and found the lung cancer.

As of that day, Doug couldn't drive. I'd been doing child care in our home, but he couldn't handle the uproar of the kids. I had to call all my customers and tell them not to come anymore.

—Carol (Doug's wife)

A person who has lung cancer must endure uncomfortable symptoms and difficult medical procedures. You, as a caregiver, are spared the physical suffering—but you share the emotional anguish. In addition, you assume many new burdens, from increased domestic responsibilities, to financial worries, to the many extra tasks associated with caregiving. Some of your chores may be scary or unpleasant, such as giving injections or providing bedpans. The person with lung cancer is your spouse, your mother or father, or your close friend. Now your role may be more like that of a parent. And the person you knew so well may be significantly altered by the disease.

In a very real way, cancer has struck you too. Yet as everyone rallies to help the patient, few offer assistance or sympathy to you. When I talk to lung cancer caregivers, I often worry that they're not getting the support they need and that they're not taking good care of themselves. That's why we wanted this book to include a chapter just for you.

———

When I have chemo, my husband is at my side. It's never "I" or "you." He says, "We have a CT scan on Friday."
—Donna P.

———

Coping with the Challenge

Caregiving is very stressful work. A study published in *Social Science and Medicine* in 2000 found that when couples faced cancer, it was the spouse, not the patient, who suffered the most emotional distress. What's more, spouses received less support from others. But there was also good news from the study: over time, both partners adjusted to the diagnosis. Here are a few suggestions for speeding the process:

Communicate as Openly as Possible

When someone you love is seriously ill and going through difficult treatment, the last thing you want to do is to add to the misery. So you may try to conceal your own anguish. The result, despite your good intentions, can be painful misunderstanding. Donna M.—who now describes her husband's loving support as "the reason I have made it this far"—recalls the upsetting period shortly after her diagnosis, when she was still recovering from surgery:

I'd be in bed. My husband would be in the hallway cleaning out the closets. He was keeping himself busy because he was hurting so, but I didn't know that. I felt he was cleaning me out. I didn't share these feelings until we went to see my oncologist. I started crying and we cried together for the first time. It was the beginning of a growing time for us that is still happening.

Many people facing lung cancer discover that expressing their thoughts, even the upsetting ones, brings new intimacy to their relationship. But you may find yourself in a situation where frank discussion is particularly difficult. For example, the patient may be unwilling to face a bleak prognosis. Or his personality may be altered by the disease or by treatment. Carol, whom you met at the beginning of this chapter, says of her husband, Doug, who was treated for brain metastases:

There have been a lot of mental changes. He's forgetful and that will never come back. He's bad-tempered, and thinks he's right.

If you and the patient find it difficult to talk to each other about important issues, a third person—such as a close friend, a doctor, or a counselor—might be able to help. Ben and his wife went for couples counseling for about six months after his diagnosis. He had just been diagnosed with stage IV disease; they had two young children, ages 3 and 5. On top of everything else, they had recently moved back into a remodeled house that they were trying to put into order. Says Ben:

It's harder on the caretaker than the patient. My wife had all kinds of responsibilities to think about. The counselor facilitated her ability to express her fears openly, which helped us communicate better.

Don't Try to Do It All

Caregiving responsibilities come as additions to what is probably already a full schedule. Your first impulse may be to try to stretch yourself, doing everything you did before plus all the new extras. But you need to conserve your energy, for the patient's sake as well as for yourself.

Cut Back

Many of us chronically try to do too much. We spend too many hours at work; we try to cram too much into our days. Or we get locked into particu-

When Other Family Members Don't Do Their Fair Share

If you're struggling to help a person with lung cancer, it's frustrating when other family members don't contribute nearly as much. Sometimes they actually make additional demands instead of helping out. Here are recommendations:

- **Share information.** Keep the rest of the family up-to-date about the patient's medical news and other pertinent developments.

- **Ask directly for what you need.** You may assume that needs are obvious, but they may not be. Other family members may be preoccupied with their own lives; or they may be waiting to be asked for fear of intruding.

- **Call a family conference.** It's much better to raise the subject before you become angry. If you already feel angry, try to resolve your emotions ahead of time: your goal is to draw family members closer, but anger will push them away. Think about what you will say. Consider practicing with a trusted friend, a counselor, or a caregiver support group. If necessary, ask a professional—such as a doctor, oncology nurse, social worker, or religious adviser—to help you talk to family members.

- **Adjust your expectations.** Even if other family members do much less than you do (and much less than you feel they should), their contributions are still valuable. If you express appreciation they're more likely to do more in the future.

- **Seek help outside the family.** Family members may be willing to pay for additional services if they can't assist themselves.

lar ways of doing things, even if they're inefficient. Now that you're a caregiver, there are even more demands on your time. If you don't cut back, you may become exhausted or find yourself unable to meet important responsibilities. A few recommendations:

- Tell your employer, your family, and others how your life has changed and what your limitations are. Ask them to reduce what they expect of you.

- Delegate responsibilities as much as possible. You may be reluctant to impose. Or perhaps you feel that others won't handle the tasks properly and that it's easier to do it yourself than to teach and supervise. These are reasonable concerns, but you need to get past them.

- Set priorities. If some tasks must go undone, it's better to decide which these will be. Ask yourself what is truly important and what can be omitted.

Get Help

Hiring help or paying for services can lighten your load. Unfortunately, lung cancer often means that your financial resources are limited too. Find out if you're eligible for assistance from your insurer or your community (see

Signs of Caregiver Burnout

Here are signs that caregiving is having a negative effect on your physical and emotional health:

- **Anger and hostility:** Overreacting to minor frustrations or saying things you regret to the patient, family members, friends, medical caregivers, or others

- **Depression:** Continuing to feel low-spirited and hopeless rather than adjusting to the diagnosis after a few months; being unable to enjoy activities that used to give you pleasure, such as spending time with family or friends

- **Other emotional reactions that are unusual for you:** Crying more easily or feeling particularly fearful or anxious

- **Mental changes:** Becoming forgetful or unable to concentrate

- **Changes in eating and drinking:** Eating a lot more and gaining

Chapter 19). For example, your health care coverage might include visits by a home health aide while the patient is recovering from surgery.

Asking for help from friends and relatives isn't easy. And even when assistance is offered, you may find it difficult to accept. Some suggestions:

- Realize that people who care about you genuinely want to contribute. Grant them the blessing of acting generously.

- Be prepared with answers to the question "What can I do to help?" Make a list of tasks, from shopping and laundry, to driving children to activities, to bathing a patient who is bedridden at home. If many chores and helpers are involved, ask someone to be in charge of scheduling everything.

- Set realistic standards. Some jobs will be done badly or differently from how you normally do them. Unless the problem is truly significant—for instance, something that endangers the patient—let it go.

---

weight, or losing interest in food and eating inadequately; drinking more alcohol than usual

- **Sleep disturbances:** Being unable to fall asleep or waking up too early; sleeping poorly so you don't feel rested in the morning

- **Exhaustion:** Feeling tired all the time, despite getting enough sleep

- **Nagging health problems:** Headaches, upset stomach, or new aches and pains

If you recognize that you're suffering from burnout, resolve to help yourself:

- Delegate the most onerous caregiving responsibilities, at least temporarily, even if it means that you must impose on others or pay more than you can really afford.

- Join a support group for caregivers (see Resources on pages 312–313).

- Seek professional help from a psychologist, social worker, religious adviser, or other counselor.

Take Care of Yourself

As your "to do" list lengthens, it will become harder to find time for yourself. But you need to be nurtured and replenished to be able to give fully to your loved one. These ideas may help:

- Find things to do and talk about that don't involve cancer. Maintain your own interests and friendships.

- Schedule time off instead of hoping that free time will materialize. It won't. Also, take as many mini-breaks as possible. For example, if your loved one has a medical appointment and you're facing a long wait, go for a walk or call a friend to talk.

- Develop a support network. Reach out to friends; join a support group for caregivers (see Resources below). Carol says:

  I have wonderful girlfriends. During the first year after Doug was diagnosed, I was on the phone every day with them. They listened to me for hours and hours and hours.

- Don't neglect your own health. That means taking time for exercise (even if it's just a short walk) and for regular meals, as well as for medical checkups.

Resources

The books and brochures we've suggested throughout the book for lung cancer patients are helpful for caregivers too. Here are additional materials that provide insights and practical advice:

- *Taking Time: Support for People with Cancer and the People Who Care About Them*, a free booklet from the National Cancer Institute (*http://www. cancer.gov/cancerinfo/takingtime* or call 800-4-CANCER).

- *Caregiving: A Step-by-Step Resource for Caring for the Person with Cancer at Home*, by Peter S. Houts and Julia A. Bucher (American Cancer Society, 2000). Available at bookstores or order from ACS (800-ACS-2345).

Most cancer patient support groups welcome caregivers. But caregivers may be able to speak more freely in a group of their own. Use the following resources plus those listed on page 137 to locate an appropriate group:

- The ALCASE hotline (800-298-2436) provides support to caregivers as well as to patients. The ALCASE Phone Buddy service can connect caregivers to others in a similar situation.

- Cancer Care's web site includes a special section for caregivers (*http://www.cancercare.org/CaregiverResources*) with advice on everything from coping with treatment side effects to workplace issues for people who need to take time off to care for a loved one. Cancer Care's telephone support is available to caregivers too (800-813-HOPE).

- ACOR (Association of Cancer Online Resources) hosts several online discussion groups for caregivers of people with cancer (*http://listserv .acor.org/archives/caregivers.html*).

- Well Spouse Foundation (800-838-0879; *http://www.wellspouse.org*) is a national organization that provides support to spouses and partners of people who are chronically ill or disabled.

- *Today's Caregiver* is a bimonthly magazine for all caregivers. Call 800-829-2734 or see Caregiver.com (*http://www.caregiver.com*) for a subscription; the web site also offers a free newsletter, online discussion groups, and information.

- National Family Caregivers Association is an advocacy organization for people who care for chronically ill, aged, or disabled loved ones (800-896-3650; *http://www.nfcacares.org*).

Caregiving for a loved one with lung cancer may be one of the toughest jobs that will confront you in your lifetime. However—and this will sound odd—it can also be one of the most rewarding. The person with lung cancer is someone already very close to you. Now both of you are terribly vulnerable, faced with a life-threatening illness. You have an opportunity to get to know each other more deeply than ever before. You also may see yourself in a new way. Caregiving requires strength you might not know you had. May you take great pride in all you are accomplishing, and cherish the special memories and insights that caregiving brings.

The Practicalities

I was self-employed—and overnight I can't produce an income. We had to sell my truck and our two cars to save our house. Financially, we were destroyed. But out of nowhere, people came around to help. Friends, acquaintances, neighbors all showed up with money and food, anything they could do. I'll never forget that.
—Doug

———

When you're diagnosed with lung cancer, your health is your first concern. But practical matters follow close behind: insurance, your job, your finances. You quickly learn that medical expertise is not the only kind you need. How well you deal with your insurance company or HMO, with your employer, and with creditors can make a difference in the quality of your medical care—and in the quality of your life.

This chapter discusses these practicalities. We can't cover everything, but we'll help you get started and point you to helpful resources. You'll be relieved to see how much is available. You are not alone.

Dealing with Insurance, Managed Care, and HMOs

We hope you're fortunate enough to have health insurance when cancer strikes. (If not, skip to the box on page 318.) Consider yourself doubly blessed if your plan is a source of support and security. Unfortunately, not all are. And even the best insurers have rules and procedures that you'll need to follow.

Many people don't get everything they're entitled to from their health insurance. They may not realize what's covered; or they may feel so over-whelmed (or intimidated) that they don't make claims, don't correct mistakes, and don't appeal adverse decisions. Here are suggestions for becoming a savvy insurance consumer:

Understand Your Coverage

Read the fine print. Ask for help if you find the policy lengthy and confusing (see box on page 321 on getting help with insurance problems). Don't delay. The information could affect the quality of your care or the amount you will have to pay yourself. Here are relevant issues:

- What's covered? Before you agree to tests or treatment, find out if they're covered by your insurance.

- What procedures must be followed to obtain coverage for the care you need? For example, the insurer may require you to have a referral from your primary care physician before you can see a specialist; a second opinion may be necessary for coverage of surgery. If you're in an HMO or managed care plan, coverage may be limited to particular doctors and hospitals.

Are You a Veteran?

The Veteran's Health Administration (VHA) provides a broad range of medical services—including hospitalization, prescription drugs, and rehabilitation—to many men and women who served in the U.S. military. Some veterans don't realize that they are entitled to assistance under current rules. For information about eligibility requirements and benefits, contact the Department of Veterans Affairs (800-827-1000) or visit the VA web site: *http://www.va.gov.*

Staying Covered

When you have cancer, it's more important than ever to maintain your health insurance coverage. Usually this is possible, though the cost of your insurance may go up and your benefits may be reduced after the diagnosis.

- Pay your insurance bills on time.

- Get expert advice before changing insurance plans and before making any change in your life that could affect your insurance. That includes leaving your job (or your spouse leaving his or her job) if you're insured through an employer; it even includes getting divorced if you're insured via your spouse.

- If you're insured through work and must leave your job, talk to your employer's benefits counselor about your options. You may be able to convert your group insurance to an individual plan.

- What must you do to obtain medical help in an emergency? If you're away from home?

- Is there a deductible? A cap on benefits?

- What are the rules concerning renewal of the policy?

- How can the insurer's decisions be appealed?

Keep Complete Records

We've already discussed the importance of keeping good medical records. It's equally important to stay on top of insurance and billing paperwork. Otherwise you may wind up paying much more than you should. Record keeping is simpler if you're in an HMO.

Managing billing records and filing insurance claims can be draining. Ask for help (see box on page 321) if you need it. At the very least, set up a single place—an accordion file, a drawer, or even a laundry basket or carton

Two federal laws provide some protection to people who might otherwise lose health benefits:

- **COBRA** (Consolidated Omnibus Reconciliation Act) may allow you to temporarily keep group health insurance obtained from an employer if you lose your job. If coverage was through your spouse, COBRA may permit continuation coverage if your spouse dies or you get divorced. You must pay for this insurance; often the cost is greater than before because you pay both your share and the employer's share of the premium. The Pension and Welfare Benefits Administration of the U.S. Department of Labor offers more information (800-998-7542; *http://www.dol.gov/dol/topic/health-plans/cobra.htm*).

- **HIPAA** (Health Insurance Portability and Accountability Act) offers limited protections if you already have health insurance but are threatened with the loss of benefits. For information, call the Centers for Medicare and Medicaid Services at 877-267-2323 or visit *http://cms.hhs.gov/hipea*. Or contact your state insurance department (see state government listings in your telephone directory).

—as a catch-all for medical and insurance papers. If everything is in one spot, it will be much easier to locate records even if they aren't organized. Here are items to file and keep:

- Your insurance policy and any amendments.

- Correspondence with your insurer, doctors, hospitals, and social agencies.

- Summaries of relevant conversations. Include the date and time, as well as the name, title, and telephone number of the person you spoke with. Send a copy of the summary to the person you spoke with, so you'll both have the same record.

- Statements from your insurer.

- Bills and receipts for payments.

- Records of travel and other expenses related to your medical care, which may be tax-deductible.

Check Charges and Statements

Billing mistakes are common—and they can be expensive. Here's how to stay on top of medical services and charges:

- Keep a diary of all medical services you receive, including tests and doctor visits, whether you're treated in your doctor's office or in the hospital.

- Get receipts for any payments you make.

- Compare your diary with medical bills and insurance statements. Question any discrepancies promptly. Request new bills or statements if you find mistakes. Review those too, to make sure mistakes were corrected.

If You're Not Insured

Forty-four million Americans have no health insurance. If you're among them, getting good medical care will be a challenge—but it *is* possible.

- Talk to your doctor and work out a manageable payment plan. Most doctors are sympathetic to financially strapped patients. Your doctor may be able to refer you to programs offering free or subsidized assistance, such as clinical trials that cover expenses or drug company programs that provide medication at no cost.

- Talk with a social worker or patient advocate at the hospital where you're being treated. Ask for help in negotiating a less onerous payment schedule and for suggestions about other resources.

- Find out if you're eligible for Medicaid, a federal and state program that pays for the medical care of people with low incomes. Call the Centers for Medicare and Medicaid Services for information (800-633-4227).

- Call local or national cancer advocacy groups for advice, such as ALCASE (800-298-2436), the American Cancer Society (800-ACS-2345), or Cancer Care (800-813-HOPE).

- See other suggestions throughout this chapter.

If It's Not Covered by Insurance, Perhaps It's Tax-Deductible

Even the best insurance doesn't cover all out-of-pocket expenses for medical care. But Uncle Sam may be able to help on April 15, depending on the nature of the expense as well as your income and how you file your taxes. See Internal Revenue Service Publication 502, *Medical and Dental Expenses*, available from the IRS web site (*http://www.irs.gov*) or your local IRS office (check federal government listings in your telephone directory).

- Document your efforts to correct errors. Keep a telephone log and copies of correspondence.

Appeal If Necessary

What if you need treatment that your insurer refuses to cover, or your insurer denies a claim that you believe should be paid? Some insurance companies try to save money by covering only older, less expensive treatments. They may define as "experimental" a treatment that your doctor regards as standard—for instance, a chemotherapy drug that has FDA approval for a different type of cancer, but that many doctors are successfully using to treat lung cancer. Or they may resist your attempts to see a specialist.

Nearly all health insurers have a process for appealing their decisions. If you know your rights, you have a good chance of succeeding.

- Review the rules and check your records so you can make the best possible case for yourself.

- Talk to your doctor. Sometimes a call or letter from your doctor can make the difference between yes and no. For instance, your doctor can explain that your treatment is, in fact, consistent with current practices.

- Write to the insurance company. Effective letters state the facts succinctly, clearly, and politely. Also useful is a letter from your doctor or a copy of a relevant medical article. (Read sample letters on the web site of the

Patient Advocate Foundation: *http://www.patientadvocate.org.*) Send your letter via certified mail or a delivery service so you can prove that it arrived.

- If your appeal is denied, try again. Insurers usually provide more than one level of appeal. You also can appeal outside the plan if necessary. If you're on Medicare, call the Medicare hotline (800-633-4227) for information. Otherwise, call your state insurance commissioner (see state government listings in your telephone directory) to learn if you have any recourse. Some states have provisions for external review of certain insurance decisions.

Insurance Information Resources

The following provide helpful written materials and other assistance regarding insurance companies and HMOs:

- State insurance commissioners (see state government listing in your local telephone directory)

- The Georgetown University Institute for Health Care Research and Policy web site (*http://www.healthinsuranceinfo.net*) offers state-specific versions of a brochure titled *A Consumer Guide for Getting and Keeping Health Insurance.*

- The National Coalition for Cancer Survivorship sells publications that cover insurance issues, including a booklet called *What Cancer Survivors*

What's the Billing Code?

Medical procedures—everything from drawing blood to removing a lung—are coded for insurance purposes. Payment may be less than it should be simply because the procedure was coded one way rather than another, or because the wrong code was assigned.

Codes are listed on the printout you'll receive from your insurer. If a procedure isn't covered fully, talk to the person in charge of billing at your doctor's office. Ask if the code is correct, or if there's another way to code the procedure to obtain better coverage.

Getting Help with Insurance Problems

If you feel overwhelmed by medical paperwork and insurance red tape, find someone to assist you. The sooner you take charge, the more quickly those ominous paper piles will disappear and the more easily problems will be solved.

- Ask a trusted friend or relative to spend a few hours a week catching up with your paperwork—someone who isn't intimidated by complicated rules and financial calculations.

- Hire an accountant, bookkeeper, or financial adviser—preferably one familiar with medical record keeping. Ask about prices. If ongoing help would be too expensive, schedule a single session to set up a simple-to-use filing system you can manage on your own.

- Call a community service organization or private company that handles medical paperwork. Get a referral from a patient support group or from a hospital or community social worker or patient advocate.

If you need help appealing a decision, contact any or all of the following:

- Your insurance agent or the personnel office of your employer (or your spouse's employer) if insurance is through work

- Your doctor or your doctor's office manager; a social worker, patient advocate, or financial counselor at the hospital where you're treated

- Your state insurance commissioner's office (see state government listings in your local telephone directory)

- The Patient Advocate Foundation, a nonprofit organization that helps patients resolve insurance and other financial problems regarding health care (800-532-5274; *http://www.patientadvocate .org*)

Can I Get Health Insurance Now, Even if I've Had Cancer?

After cancer, health insurance usually becomes harder to obtain, and more expensive. There may be special waiting periods and other restrictions because of your medical history. But it's not impossible.

- Purchase insurance through a group, such as your employer, your spouse's employer, or a professional or fraternal organization.

- Contact your state insurance commissioner for other options (check telephone book under state government). Some states require HMOs to have open enrollment periods in which they accept anyone who applies, regardless of medical history, or they may have a high-risk pool for people who can't get insurance through normal channels.

- Find out if you're eligible for Medicare (which covers most people age 65 and over as well as those who are permanently disabled) or Medicaid (which covers people with low income; eligibility varies by state). For information, call your local Social Security Administration office (see federal government listings in your telephone directory).

- Consider joining a religious medical cost-sharing plan, in which monthly membership fees are used to pay participants' medical expenses. One example is the Christian Brotherhood Newsletter (330-848-1511; *http://www.christianbrotherhood.org*); your religious counselor may know of similar organizations. These plans typically have less stringent requirements than traditional insurers concerning preexisting conditions, but very strict standards regarding religious observance and lifestyle. Also note that these plans usually are not regulated by the state laws that govern conventional insurance companies.

Need to Know about Health Insurance. Call or visit their web site (877-NCCS-YES; *http://www.canceradvocacy.org*).

• The Patient Advocate Foundation provides informative booklets about insurance on its web site (*http://www.patientadvocate.org*; click on "Resources"); some are available in print form. Call 800-532-5274 to order materials or to ask questions about insurance.

• The American Association of Retired Persons (AARP) provides free brochures on Medicare and on other health insurance options for people age 50 and up (800-424-3410; *http://www.aarp.org*).

Can I Still Get Life Insurance?

Not surprisingly, it's difficult to purchase life insurance after a lung cancer diagnosis. If you need life insurance to provide for loved ones who depend on your income, consider the possibilities below. Before you make a decision, read the terms very carefully. An independent insurance agent, who is familiar with policies from many companies, may be able to help you.

• A group plan from your employer or an organization to which you belong. Sometimes these don't require a medical history or physical examination.

• A policy from a company that specializes in high-risk life insurance. Such policies are expensive.

• A policy with limited benefits (called a graded policy). Medical information may not be requested, but death benefits depend on how long you survive after you purchase the policy.

• Guaranteed life insurance that requires no medical history or physical examination. These policies are usually costly and beneficiaries can't collect the full face value unless you survive at least one year or perhaps longer.

• Mortgage or credit card insurance, which could pay these debts in the event of your death. These policies may not require medical information.

- The National Cancer Institute's free brochure *Facing Forward: A Guide for Cancer Survivors* includes a useful section on insurance. It's available online (*http://www.cancer.gov/cancerinfo/life-after-treatment*) or by calling 800-4-CANCER.

- The web site of the Health Insurance Association of America, a trade association representing the private health care system, offers basic brochures about health insurance as well as a state-by-state list of addresses and phone numbers for free state or federally funded insurance counseling (*http://www.hiaa.org*).

Making a Living

In Chapter 9 we discussed the period right after your diagnosis, when you tell your employer that you have lung cancer (see pages 132–133). What happens afterward? Much depends on your preferences. Perhaps you enjoy your work and your colleagues—or maybe you need the money and benefits, including health insurance. On the other hand, you might decide it's time for a change, and seek another job or retire.

If You Want to Return to Work

Develop a tentative plan. You may be able to work full-time or part-time during and immediately after treatment, or you might need to take several weeks off. Review your benefits package to learn about sick leave and other personal leave policies. Also talk to your doctor and to other lung cancer survivors to find out how you're likely to feel during and after treatment. Of course, your responses won't be exactly the same as other people's. However, your experience generally will be quite different from that of someone with breast, prostate, or other cancer that does not affect a vital organ.

If you'd like to continue with your job after treatment, consider what it would take to make that possible. Begin by talking informally to the people at work whose support you'll need, such as your immediate supervisor or the personnel office. Follow up discussions with a letter or memo summarizing any agreements made to accommodate you. Your employer and colleagues may be very supportive. However, surveys suggest that about 25 percent of cancer survivors encounter discrimination. According to the National Coali-

Legal Protections for Cancer Patients

Federal and state laws protect cancer patients, though not every employee is covered. To find out what protections apply to you, contact the civil rights or human rights agency in your state (see state government listings in your telephone directory). Three important federal laws:

- **The Americans with Disabilities Act (ADA)** prohibits some forms of discrimination against people with cancer who are capable of performing the essential functions of a job. For more information about the law, contact the U.S. Equal Employment Opportunity Commission (800-669-4000; *http://www.eeoc.gov*).

- **The Family and Medical Leave Act (FMLA)** requires some employers to permit workers to take unpaid leave for their own or a family member's medical treatment. For more information about FMLA, call the U.S. Department of Labor's Wage and Hour Division (look for the Department of Labor federal government listings in your local telephone directory), or visit *http://www.dol.gov/dol/esa/fmla.htm.*

- **The Health Insurance Portability and Accountability Act (HIPAA)** was expanded in 2003 to include patient privacy provisions, which protect the confidentiality of health information. For information, call 866-627-7748 or visit *http://www.hhs.gov/ocr/hipaa.*

tion for Cancer Survivorship, the most commonly reported problems include dismissal, denial of promotion, undesirable transfer, and hostility in the workplace.

Try to use your employer's existing mechanisms to resolve any difficulties. Ask your doctor to reassure your boss about your capabilities. Other sources of assistance are colleagues, your union, medical social workers, and advocacy groups. Keep written records of your efforts to deal with the situation, as well as the responses from your employer.

I'm a lawyer, and I work at a small law firm. They were terrific. They hooked me up with a computer at home, so I stayed in touch with clients to the extent that I could. Other lawyers took over most of my cases so I didn't have a big caseload.
—Ben

Resources If You Need Help with Your Employer

Cancer support groups can provide a simple overview of your rights, as well as referrals for further assistance. If informal persuasion and routine problem-solving procedures don't work, you may have remedies under state and federal laws (see box on page 325). Since the laws have filing deadlines, explore these possibilities promptly if you think you will need them.

- The National Coalition for Cancer Survivorship (NCCS) answers questions about employment rights and provides assistance locating legal resources. Its booklets include *Working It Out: Your Employment Rights as a Cancer Survivor* (877-NCCS-YES; *http://www.cansearch.org*).

- Cancer Care's web site (*http://www.cancercare.org*) has valuable information on dealing with workplace issues. Its toll-free counseling line, which is staffed by oncology social workers, can answer questions and connect you with local resources: 800-813-HOPE.

- The National Cancer Institute's Cancer Information Service can answer questions about employment concerns. Call 800-4-CANCER to talk to a cancer information specialist or to order NCI's free booklet *Facing Forward: A Guide for Cancer Survivors*, which includes a chapter on job issues. Online, *http://www.cancer.gov/cancerinfo/life-after-treatment*.

- The Job Accommodation Network, a service of the President's Committee on Employment of People with Disabilities, can work with you and your employer to find reasonable ways to accommodate your needs (800-526-7234; *http://janweb.icdi.wvu.edu*).

- For state-level assistance with your employer, check your telephone directory's state government listings for resources on discrimination, affirmative action, or labor.

If You Can't Work at Your Previous Job

Lung cancer may make it impossible for you to continue the work you did before. Depending on your circumstances and preferences, you may decide to retrain for another career, go on disability, or take early retirement. Consider your options carefully; it's helpful to talk to a job counselor, a benefits specialist, or a financial planner.

Vocational Rehabilitation

Each state has a vocational rehabilitation agency; services may include testing and counseling, training, and job placement—as well as financial assistance. For information, contact the local office of the Social Security Administration (see telephone directory), or talk to social workers in community service programs or your hospital.

Disability

If you're unable to continue working at any job, you may qualify for disability payments. Some employee benefits packages include disability insurance, or you may have purchased this kind of insurance on your own. Check to see if you have such a policy and, if so, what provisions it contains.

Another possibility, if you're under age 65, is Social Security disability benefits. For information about eligibility requirements, contact your local Social Security office (see federal government listings in your telephone directory), or call 800-772-1213 or visit the Social Security web site (*http://www.ssa.gov*).

▬

I'm on Social Security disability. I work a little part-time each week, but I no longer have the stamina or the strength to maintain a job. I get mentally tired and I'm done. My short-term memory is history. Because of the damage to my brain, that won't ever improve.
—Doug

▬

Retirement

Depending on your age, your financial situation, and your preferences, retirement may be an option if lung cancer impairs your ability to work. Get expert advice to help you decide what's right for you, since the options can be complicated and the stakes are high.

———

I couldn't prove that contamination from the building caused my cancer, but it was definitely a source of stress. My doctor wrote letters on my behalf, but he wouldn't say that the building caused my cancer. My employer let me work at another site for three months. After that they wanted me to return to my old building. I said, "I'm not going back there."

At the time I was going through chemotherapy. I just didn't have the strength to fight, so I decided to retire on disability. When I filed my application at the Social Security office they asked me, "Why didn't you apply six months ago? You're entitled; you've paid into the system since you were sixteen years old." I knew I was fortunate to be able to take early retirement at age 56, but there were tears in my eyes. My work meant everything to me; it was my whole identity.
—Joyce

———

Your Finances

Worry about money may rival your fears about the disease. Expenses are up while income is down or less certain. If your partner is taking time off from work to help you, his or her income may be affected too. Money problems can balloon if they're ignored and some solutions require time to activate, so act promptly.

Take Stock

Look at the future as well as the present. When decisions are complex—for instance, whether you should borrow money against your house or cash in a retirement account—professional advice can be very helpful. A financial plan can help you set priorities and maximize the resources available to you.

How to Find a Financial Planner

Request recommendations from friends, your accountant or attorney, or from financial specialists at your work or in your union or other professional organization. Ask prospective planners about their qualifications and experience working with people in your situation. Find out what the service will cost and who is paying for it. Some planners earn all or part of their money from commissions, which may bias their advice. For additional information and referrals, contact the following organizations:

• The Certified Financial Planner Board of Standards (CFP Board) certifies financial planners. See its web site (*http://www.cfp.net*) for information, including a financial planning kit with advice on selecting and working with a planner. For a referral to a CFP practitioner, contact the Financial Planning Association: 800-282-PLAN.

• The National Association of Personal Financial Advisors (NAPFA), an association of fee-only planners (financial planners who do not earn money from commissions), provides referrals (888-FEE-ONLY; *http://www.napfa.org*).

Make the Most of Your Assets

Lung cancer is the proverbial rainy day. You may have dipped into your savings already. If that's not enough, you may be looking at the money tied up in investments, your home, your retirement accounts, or your life insurance policies. Be careful! You want to get the most out of these valuable resources without compromising the future financial security of you and your family. Seek expert advice before you act. And always compare prices when you shop for loans or financial settlements. Buying money is just like any other consumer purchase: prices may vary considerably and it pays to look around for the best deal.

If You Can't Pay the Bills

If you're running out of cash to pay bills, talk to creditors immediately. Or ask one of the credit counseling organizations listed below to do it for you. Most creditors—including banks, credit card companies, landlords, utilities, doctors, and hospitals—will work out a reasonable payment schedule. That takes the pressure off you and reassures them that they'll be paid eventually.

- The National Foundation for Credit Counseling (NFCC) is a national nonprofit network that advises people in stressful financial situations. Services include managing debt repayment: NFCC makes arrangements with creditors on your behalf, often including reduced or waived financial charges; you pay a manageable amount each month, which NFCC distributes to pay your bills. For information, visit its web site (*http://www.nfcc.org*) or call 800-388-2227.

- Myvesta.org, a nonprofit Internet-based organization, offers debt repayment services. For information, call 800-680-3328 or visit its web site (*http://www.myvesta.org*), which provides helpful free information about money and debt management.

If You Need Financial Help

Asking for money isn't easy. You may feel ashamed or worried about being turned down. These painful burdens are exacerbated by lengthy, confusing applications. And meanwhile you're dealing with a life-threatening illness.

Nevertheless, we hope you'll find the strength to ask for what you need. When money problems are eased, you can focus on your health. Getting back on your feet financially means that you're less of a burden to others. In time, you may be able to help other people just as you were helped.

For an overview of community help sources, see the National Cancer Institute's free brochure *How to Find Resources in Your Own Community If You Have Cancer* (800-4-CANCER; *http://cis.nci.nih.gov/fact/8-9.htm*).

Government Services

Find out if you're entitled to federal, state, or local assistance, which takes the form of money or services.

- Supplemental Security Income (SSI), which pays monthly benefits, is available to individuals with limited resources who are disabled or age 65 or older. If you qualify for SSI, you may also be eligible for food stamps, Medicaid, and other government aid. For more information, see the Social Security web site (*http://www.ssa.gov/pubs/11000.html* has information on SSI), visit your local Social Security office, or call the Social Security Administration (800-772-1213).

- Talk to your state and local social service department (listed in the telephone directory under state and local government). If you're disabled or over age 60, you may qualify for services for the elderly. Call state and local government agencies or administrations on aging. Another useful information resource is a hospital social worker or a cancer support group.

Researching Help Options

Finding the right resources can take some effort. A friend or family member may be willing to do the research for you. To keep organized, record relevant information in a notebook, including the names of people you speak with and the dates of your conversations.

Here are questions to ask:

- Am I eligible for this assistance?

- What help is provided?

- What must I do to apply? What documents and information are needed?

- When can I expect a response to my application? How long does it take for assistance to begin?

- Do you know of any other programs that might be useful?

Community Services

Civic and religious organizations may provide financial or other assistance for people with cancer. If you're disabled or over age 60, you may qualify for additional help.

- If you belong to a religious organization—such as a church, synagogue, or mosque—ask for its assistance. In addition to money, it may be able to provide transportation, housekeeping, meals, and companionship.

- Contact the local chapter of the American Cancer Society or the local United Way to ask about services in your community (see telephone directory).

- Explore the Yellow Pages of your telephone directory. Headings to check include "Community Organizations," "Human Service Organizations," and "Social Service Organizations."

Personal Fund-raising

In time of need, caring friends and family members may open their wallets to help out. This can be done informally if the amounts are small, though it never hurts to put your understandings in writing. But if you're receiving large sums of money, formalize your agreement and consider tax consequences. For example, under current law a gift over $10,000 can trigger gift tax if you are the recipient—but there's no limit for payments made directly to a medical provider on your behalf. If you receive a loan at a below-market rate, the Internal Revenue Service may consider it a gift even if you're expected to pay it back. To avoid problems, get advice from a lawyer or accountant who is familiar with the relevant issues.

Some cancer patients, faced with enormous bills, have publicized their plight within their community to raise money or have held fund-raising events. If you're considering this option, get advice from an officer at your bank. Other resources:

- The Philanthropic Advisory Service of the Council of Better Business Bureaus has a useful free publication titled *CBBB Standards for Charitable Solicitations* (703-276-0100; *http://www.give.org/standards*).

- A helpful book is *Successful Fundraising: A Complete Handbook for Volunteers and Professionals*, by Joan Flanagan (Contemporary Books, 1999).

Additional Assistance for Cancer Patients

The programs below provide cancer patients with free or low-cost transportation, lodgings, and drugs. Some are available to all; others are just for those in financial need. For additional resources, see Cancer Care's free publication *A Helping Hand: The Resource Guide for People with Cancer*, which lists hundreds of regional and national nonprofit organizations (800-813-HOPE; *http://www.cancercare.org*).

Local Travel

If driving is difficult, friends and family members may be able to assist. Here are other options:

- The American Cancer Society has a service program called "Road to Recovery," available in some locations, in which volunteers drive qualified patients to and from treatment. Call your local ACS office.

- Some communities offer low-cost door-to-door transportation for the disabled. Check with your local public transportation department and agencies for the elderly.

- A local civic or religious organization may offer volunteer drivers.

Long-Distance Travel

If you need to travel to another location for cancer treatment or consultations, expenses can mount—especially if a family member accompanies you. These programs might help:

- The National Patient Travel Center facilitates patient access to charitable medical air transportation programs for people in financial need, including private pilot volunteers, corporate airlift programs, and reduced-cost or free services from commercial airlines (800-296-1217; *http://www.patienttravel.org*).

- AirLifeLine is a charitable organization of private pilots who donate their services to patients who can't afford travel for medical care (877-AIRLIFE; *http://www.airlifeline.org*).

- The Corporate Angel Network provides free air transportation on corporate aircraft with empty seats for patients traveling to cancer centers for treatment; they do not require that you show financial need (914-328-1313; *http://www.corpangelnetwork.org*).

Accommodations

Ask a social worker at the distant hospital about any special programs or discounts for accommodations. Think about the groups you belong to. You may be able to find volunteer hosts via a religious, alumni, union, professional, fraternal, or hobby organization. Other possibilities:

- The National Association of Hospital Hospitality Houses unites more than 150 nonprofit organizations that provide lodging for families whose loved ones are receiving medical treatment far from home (800-542-9730; *http://www.nahhh.org*).

- The American Cancer Society's Hope Lodges provide free rooms throughout the country for cancer patients and their families. You do not have to show financial need to use this service, but there are other requirements, including physician approval. For information, contact ACS at 800-ACS-2345.

Drugs

If your insurance doesn't cover prescription medications that you need but can't afford, your physician may be able to obtain them free from the manufacturer via a patient assistance program. To learn more:

- The web site of the Pharmaceutical Research and Manufacturers of America (*http://www.phrma.org*) has a searchable directory of patient prescription drug programs.

- NeedyMeds offers information about drug programs on its web site (*http://www.needymeds.com*). The same information is available in print as *The NeedyMed Manual*, but it's expensive; check to see if your local library has a copy or can order it.

- The Medicine Program does the paperwork of applying for free drug programs for uninsured patients who can show financial hardship. The service costs $5 per prescription. (573-996-7300; *http://www.TheMedi cineProgram.com*)

Taking Charge of Your Future

*After I was diagnosed, I wanted to take care of incidentals that might
affect my family afterward if I died. I had a will and trust made out
and sent a copy to each of my kids. I took pictures of my jewelry to
make sure everyone gets the right things.*
  —Anita

More than a decade later, Anita remains alive and active. Getting your
affairs in order isn't a capitulation to lung cancer; it's a way to maintain control of your life. You and your family will enjoy greater peace of mind if difficult decisions have been made and all the necessary arrangements are in
place. The first step in this process is gathering basic information.

Getting Organized

If you're like most people, your personal records—items like your birth
certificate, marriage certificate, automobile title, insurance policies, and past
income tax returns—are at least semi-organized. Probably you could find
them, but the task might challenge other family members or close friends.
Gathering these materials, and writing down what's where, will greatly help
with other tasks as you get your affairs in order.

Organizing personal records can seem like a daunting task. Here are two
resources that make it simpler:

- The National Institute on Aging offers a helpful free booklet titled *Getting
  Your Affairs in Order*, which includes a checklist. Call 800-222-2225 to order.

- *Arranging Your Financial and Legal Affairs: A Step-by-Step Guide to Getting Your Affairs in Order*, by Julie A. Calligaro (Women's Source Books
  Publishers, 1998), walks you through the process.

Making Your Wishes Known

Important decisions—about your medical care, about your family,
about your possessions—will be made at the end of your life. Unless your
wishes are known, these decisions will be made by others and your loved
ones may be troubled by uncertainty. Here are the key areas to address:

Estate Planning

Estate planning may sound like something necessary only for the wealthy. Not so. If you're married, have children, or own valuable assets such as a house or car, you need an estate plan to protect your family and your property if you die or become disabled. Two essential legal documents are:

- **Will:** A document that expresses your wishes concerning the disposition of your property and the guardianship of any minor children after your death.

- **Power of attorney:** A document that allows another person to act as your agent while you're still alive. A power of attorney can be narrow (for example, it could permit your real estate agent to sign on your behalf when you sell your house) or it can be broad enough to allow a trusted friend or relative to manage all of your affairs if you become incapacitated.

All too many people fail to make estate plans. A 1999 AARP survey of over 1,000 middle-aged and older Americans found that only 60 percent had a will. When a person dies without a will, state law determines how his or her possessions will be divided; a court decides who is in charge of the estate and what happens to minor children. In other words, if you don't make your own estate plan, your state legislature and a judge will make one for you—and the results may be very different from what you would have wanted.

You can write your own estate plan, but it's best to consult a knowledgeable attorney. Ironically, it may cost your family less to pay an attorney to draw up the necessary documents than to deal with legal expenses if you die or become incapacitated without the proper arrangements in place.

For more information on estate planning, see the web site of Nolo Press (*http://www.nolo.com*), a publisher that specializes in law books for laypeople. Two helpful books on the subject are *Estate Planning Basics*, by Denis Clifford (Nolo Press, 1999), which is brief and simple, and a more detailed version titled *Plan Your Estate: Absolutely Everything You Need to Know to Protect Your Loved Ones*, by Denis Clifford and Cora Jordan (Nolo Press, 2000).

What Do You Really Want?

When you prepare advance directives—a living will and a medical power of attorney—you confront difficult decisions about medical care at the end of life. People often say that they want to die "with dignity" or that they don't want "heroic measures" to postpone an inevitable death. But these vague descriptions don't provide the necessary specific guidance. Talk to your doctor and to the people close to you to clarify your thinking about specific issues, such as the following:

- Life-sustaining equipment to aid breathing or kidney function

- Artificial hydration (via IV) or nutrition (via tube feeding)

- CPR (cardiopulmonary resuscitation) if breathing or heartbeat stops

- Antibiotics to treat infections, such as pneumonia

- Medication to relieve physical or emotional discomfort if the medication might make you unconscious or hasten your death

Advance Directives

Advance directives allow you to guide decisions about your medical care even if you become incapacitated and can no longer communicate with your doctors. The key documents, which are not activated so long as you're able to express your wishes, are:

- **Living will**, in which you specify your preferences concerning treatment choices at the end of life. Talk to your doctor so that you understand the options.

- **Durable power of attorney for health care**, in which you name a close friend or family member to make medical decisions on your behalf if you can no longer do so. You need a medical power of attorney even if you have a living will, because it's impossible to anticipate all the decisions that must be made if you become incapacitated.

- **"Do not resuscitate" order (DNR),** an optional document used to tell your doctor and other medical personnel that you don't want to be given cardiopulmonary resuscitation (CPR) if your heartbeat or breathing stops. Please note: If you've signed a "Do not resuscitate" order, tell your family not to call 911 in an emergency; the emergency medical crew may not follow your wishes. Instead, they should call your doctor or your oncology or hospice nurse and ask for instructions.

Talk to your family about your advance directives, so they know your wishes. Make sure that your doctor and the person you entrust with your power of attorney are willing to abide by your preferences.

My mother wouldn't write a will until she was on her deathbed. She thought that would assign a date to it. It's hard to think about the end, about exactly what that disease is going to do to you. But by procrastinating, you end up thinking about it every time you procrastinate.
—*John*

Though advance directives are legal in every state, the particular forms required vary. You can obtain the necessary forms from a member of your oncology team or from these two nonprofit organizations:

- Aging with Dignity publishes *Five Wishes*, an inexpensive 12-page booklet that walks you through five key questions that cover not only end-of-life care but also funeral arrangements. *Five Wishes* can be used as a workbook for discussing relevant issues; in some states it's accepted as a legal document. For more information or to order a copy, visit the organization's web site (*http://www.agingwithdignity.org*) or call 888-5-WISHES.

- Partnership for Caring provides extensive information and how-to assistance on advance directives on its web site (*http://www.partnership forcaring.org*) and via its hotline (800-989-9455). State-specific forms are available free at the web site; printed versions can be ordered for a nominal charge.

When you have cancer, you may feel that you're fighting a war with multiple fronts. And it's true—you're up against a lot more than the disease. The sooner you tackle the practicalities, the faster you'll get them under control. Set aside a little time each day to deal with record keeping, letter writing, filing, phone calls, and the like. Ask for help if you need it. If you're a caregiver or friend, lifting this burden is one of the greatest gifts you can offer someone with lung cancer.

CHAPTER 20

It's Never Too Late to Hope

by Peggy McCarthy

I did a one-year internship as a hospital chaplain and I've worked at a hospice. So I've had a great deal of experience with death and dying. Little did I know it was preparation for today.

I've seen how to die—and how not to die. Some people aren't able to look inside themselves, for whatever reason. They struggle with letting go. But I've also seen people deal with what's given to them and handle it as best they could. At the end they were able to accept everything they've done on earth and go peacefully. Hopefully I'll be one of those.

—John

We all face death as part of being born. For most of our life, death is a far-distant event. It hardly seems real—and we'd rather not think about it. Being diagnosed with lung cancer brings death into stark reality. If you're cured or in remission, you may not want to dwell upon this possibility right now. In that case, just skim the chapter or skip to the Afterword on pages 353–354. The information will be here if you ever need it.

Increasing numbers of lung cancer survivors will die of old age or some other disease—we hope very much that you are among them. But at some point your medical team may tell you that your cancer can't be cured or controlled. You will then know that you're very likely to die from the cancer and that your remaining time is limited. Your doctors may describe the typical course of your illness, but each individual is unique. No one can tell you how long you will live.

This chapter offers information and suggestions about dealing with advanced disease based on what I've learned from people with lung cancer. With effective symptom management, they have remained comfortable until the end. Often they discover a profound sense of accomplishment and joy in their last months or weeks of life. Regardless of your present circumstances, I hope you will be relieved and encouraged by their experiences.

Finding Hope

Each phase of life offers reasons for hope. To hope means to focus on what is positive and good. Some people find that hope comes naturally, even when they're dying. Others have to work at developing these feelings. I encourage you to seek opportunities for hope, because it has great power to enrich your life.

If you have early-stage lung cancer, you will certainly hope for a cure. What is there to hope for if you have late-stage disease? Hope can take many forms. It's as individual as you are. Phil—who outlived his bleak prognosis by more than two years—focused on the milestones he hoped to reach:

> *Ten months ago my doctors said I have six months to a year. I keep setting goals for the next two or three months. In the fall, my goal was to celebrate Christmas; in the spring it was attending a bar mitzvah and my second daughter's high school graduation. My next goal is to go to France in October, after we get our daughter settled at college.*

Hope can mean bringing life to a positive conclusion by mending relationships or by learning to see the true beauty of life. Your hopes may focus on a comfortable, peaceful death. John reflects:

> *I'm a firm believer that the divine lives within all of us, and that during my life journey it's my duty to make that light shine as brightly as it can. When I was diagnosed, the radiologist said that with some good luck I'd have a year to live. From the beginning, when I got the news, I was able to say that it doesn't matter whether he's right; what matters is what I do on the journey. I prefer not to die, but that part of it I let go. Focusing on the journey keeps me from being afraid. I'm hoping it's a very peaceful and wonderful experience leaving this planet.*

There's Still Time

Unlike those who die unexpectedly, people with cancer have been given a warning. Despite their grief and sense of loss, they're often grateful for this signal. They discover that there really is time to do what matters. Tracy says:

> *Whenever I'm feeling sorry for myself, I think that somewhere in the world a mother will be killed by a car today. She'll have no time to prepare, but I have the opportunity to spend time with my daughter and create good memories. Shortly after her third birthday, I found out the cancer had recurred. A month later we went to Disney World. We talked; we laughed; we went to all the breakfasts with Disney characters. It was one of the best vacations I ever had. I try to make every day count. This doesn't mean I don't procrastinate. I want to write lots of letters to my daughter, but it's so painful that I haven't done it yet.*

Making Dreams Come True

Is there anything you've always wanted to do but have postponed? John's response to terminal illness was to enroll in school:

> *I'm not one to sit around and wring my hands about what's going to happen to me next. I went back to school to get a degree in social work. I'm taking nine credits this summer and nine credits in the fall.*

Others fulfill a lifelong desire, such as taking a special trip. Phil made an audacious purchase:

> *My daughter was driving an old car, and it died. We were planning to replace it with something similar. But I'd always wanted a sports car, so I decided to get one and give my car to my daughter. The best deal I could find was a three-year lease. I took it. I'm a lawyer and I figure no lawyer will die in a year if he's got a three-year lease.*

Drawing Closer to Loved Ones

When time is short, people often reach out to those they love. Instead of leaving thoughts and feelings unspoken, they express what is in their hearts.

Their relationships deepen and they achieve new intimacy. This is a time for creating memories to be cherished later. Glenn says:

> I want to give my girls time with me. I want them to have experiences that will allow them to remember their dad in a fun way. At the same time, I try to prepare them. I told them, "If anything happens, know that I stayed with you as long as I could. If there's any way for me to look down and help you when I'm in heaven, I will."

Understandably, these emotion-charged conversations are difficult. A communication gap can develop between people who love each other because each is trying to protect the other. Or perhaps they simply don't know what to say and feel inadequate. Try to find someone in your family with whom you can talk comfortably. Or ask a professional—a doctor, oncology nurse, therapist, social worker, hospice worker, or member of the clergy—to facilitate.

> I was diagnosed in July 1994. In the beginning, every time my husband, Jon, and I talked about the future, I started crying. That October, I was looking at pumpkins with my daughter, Jessica, who was ten. Out of the clear blue she said, "If anything happens to you, I don't want Daddy to get remarried." I forced myself to remain calm because I wanted her to feel free to talk about this. I said, "If something happens to me, I would like for him to remarry. You could help him pick out somebody really special that you like." I didn't dwell on it because I didn't want to start crying. She went right back to the pumpkins.
> —Donna P.

Finding Meaning in Life

Facing death alters how we look at life. You may ask yourself: What is life about? Why are we here? Why did this happen to me? Answers may come from religion and prayer, but traditional religion is not the only route to spirituality. Solace also may be found through reading, intimate conversation with loved ones, keeping a journal, or spending time in beautiful natural settings.

People nearing the end often find comfort in looking back on their lives. Reviewing their experiences—both the joys and the sorrows—brings a sense of meaning and closure.

━━

I've never been religious. But I've become much more receptive to the spiritual side of life. I have a faith in some being out there. This faith has grown so that I'm no longer afraid of death.
—Phil

━━

Leaving a Personal Legacy

Your memory can remain alive and you can achieve personal goals even after your death. You don't have to be wealthy to leave a rich legacy. You might want to create a journal or a family memoir. Or perhaps you'd like to write letters or record videotapes for your family and friends. Or maybe you dream of starting a special project for your community or for an organization whose work you admire.

Saying Goodbye

The people who love you will always remember your final days. You can ease their grief by telling them how much they've meant to you. Or offer a meaningful gift, such as a favorite possession that will always bring happy memories of your time together.

━━

We were sitting shoulder to shoulder, hand in hand, both of us weeping quiet tears. Chemotherapy had failed, and my beloved husband's body was overrun with cancer. "You know what hurts the worst?" he said. I waited, expecting words of grief over the future, which cancer would steal from this gentle, kind, wonderful human being. "I only have to do stage IV. But you have to do stage V. You have to stay behind. All I ever wanted was to make you happy, but I will be the cause of the greatest pain you have ever known."
—Tina

━━

Shirley Goller

Shirley Goller was diagnosed with lung cancer in 1998, and she died a year later at age 67. The disease was already advanced when it was discovered; her doctor warned that a cure was unlikely. Shirley was convinced that the cancer would have been found years earlier, in time for a cure, if lung cancer screening had been part of her routine physicals. Her son, Howard Goller, a journalist for the Reuters news agency, described her final year:

> Mom resolved to do what she could to help others escape a similar fate, even if it meant going public with experiences she might have preferred to keep private. With my support, Mom wrote an opinion piece for the Kansas City Star. She asked: If a simple mammogram could detect breast cancer and a Pap smear could locate cervical cancer, why did she have to wait until she was coughing up small blood clots? Why wasn't there a cheap, widespread method for early detection of lung cancer?
>
> Mom gave newspaper and TV interviews. We heard from four people who discovered lung cancer within weeks of reading her article. Mom filled a shoebox with letters of thanks.
>
> We had some good, long talks, and on two visits my brother and I videotaped interviews with her. When we asked Mom for advice for her grandchildren, she came up with a list of thirteen points. One seemed especially important in the context of her fight for early detection: "Be part of your community by giving."

Shirley was delighted to learn about research showing that screening for lung cancer could save lives. After her death, Howard Goller honored his mother's memory by arranging for the Reuters Foundation to sponsor an ALCASE brochure to encourage early detection of lung cancer.

Planning a Funeral or Memorial Service

Many people wouldn't want to plan the ceremony that will mark the end of their life. But those who can face this sad task give their loved ones a great gift. Even an expected death is very stressful, and so much must be accomplished right afterward. It's painful to know that you won't be there to comfort and assist. But you can help now. Planning your funeral or memorial service—listing people to invite, selecting music and readings, arranging for burial or cremation, and writing an obituary—lifts a burden from your family. Discussing these plans allows them to grieve ahead of time, while you're still able to provide loving support.

Five Wishes, a booklet published by Aging with Dignity, contains helpful discussion questions about end-of-life arrangements. For more information or to order a copy, visit the organization's web site (*http://www.agingwith dignity.org*) or call 888-5-WISHES.

A Gentle Death

Most people who die from lung cancer live through a period of days or weeks when they know that the end is near. They have a sense that the balance has tipped and the disease is taking over. Sometimes death comes suddenly, because a blood clot causes a fatal embolism, heart attack, or stroke. But usually there's a gradual but unmistakable decline in which their health and ability to care for themselves begin to fail more rapidly. Think about how you want to live through this stage before you reach it, so that you and your loved ones are prepared.

Difficult Decisions

Unlike people who die suddenly, you have the opportunity to decide how and where you want to die. If you don't yet have your affairs in order by the time your illness enters its final stage, give high priority to these tasks. (See pages 335–339 for more specific information.) If you're already prepared, review your records to be certain they reflect your current wishes. Also make sure that your doctor and loved ones support your decisions. Most people feel relieved and at peace when they know that everything is arranged.

Hospice Support

I recommend that you consider hospice for the final stage of your illness. Hospice is a team approach to end-of-life care. The team—consisting of doctors, nurses, home health aides, social workers, and religious or other counselors—provides medical and other support aimed at enhancing physical and emotional well-being as death approaches. Care may be provided in hospitals, nursing homes, or hospice facilities, but usually patients are at home. When a patient prefers to die at home, hospice can provide extensive support for caregivers to make it possible.

Hospice programs generally admit patients only when their life expectancy is six months or less. Treatments are given only for comfort, not to prolong life. However, it's best not to wait until time is very short. Indeed, I suggest that you contact your local hospice if you're diagnosed with late-stage lung cancer, even if you plan to seek aggressive treatment. That way you'll know what services are available if you need them.

Medicare and most insurance plans cover hospice services. To be eligible, your doctor usually must certify that you are terminally ill. During the period that you receive hospice care, Medicare and other insurers cover palliative (comfort-oriented) treatments, including painkillers, oxygen, and even radiation, chemotherapy, or surgery to reduce tumors causing pain or breathlessness. However, you must agree to forgo treatments aimed at curing the disease. Check with your insurer for details.

Your doctor or hospital social worker can tell you more about hospice and help you locate an appropriate program in your area. Other information resources:

- The National Hospice Foundation offers helpful information on its web site (http://*www.hospiceinfo.org*). Articles include "How to Select a Hospice Program" and "Communicating Your End of Life Wishes."

- The National Hospice and Palliative Care Organization (NHPCO) represents most U.S. hospice programs. To find an NHPCO member hospice, visit its web site (*http://www.nhpco.org*) or call its toll-free number (800-658-8898).

- Hospice Net's web site (*http://www.hospicenet.org*) has excellent information about hospice programs, as well as articles about dying and grief.

The Option of Terminal Sedation

Many patients fear a lengthy and agonizing dying process more than they fear death itself. But death from lung cancer can almost always be made peaceful and comfortable if that is your goal.

You or the person you have empowered to make your health care decisions can ask the doctor to administer whatever medication is necessary (usually narcotic painkillers and sedatives) to relieve your pain, breathlessness, or emotional agitation—even if these measures render you unconscious and might hasten your death. In addition, you or your proxy can direct that all life-extending treatments be withdrawn, including tube feeding and IV fluids. You would then sleep peacefully and painlessly until your death.

This approach, called **terminal sedation**, can be given in a hospital or hospice. Patients who prefer to die at home can receive the same medications and the same withdrawal of other treatment. Terminal sedation is legal; it's not considered assisted suicide or euthanasia. A 1997 Supreme Court decision clarified that doctors can do what's necessary to relieve suffering, even if these palliative measures shorten a patient's life, so long as the intent is to relieve suffering and not to cause death.

"But I'm Not Ready for Hospice."

Joanne called ALCASE for the first time about four years ago, shortly after she was diagnosed with lung cancer and began treatment. Over the years we spoke regularly. Last December she called to say that the cancer had begun growing again. Joanne was not a candidate for surgery or radiation—the cancer was too widespread for that; chemotherapy had been extremely difficult for her and she didn't want to try again. Joanne's physician suggested hospice. She knew her time was limited, but she said:

Hospice means I'm giving up. I might as well close my eyes and die. I'm not ready for that—there are things I want to accomplish.

Joanne and I talked for a long time. I told her that "giving up" wasn't necessarily a bad thing. She would be accepting that her disease had

Not everyone would want terminal sedation. You might prefer to endure discomfort so you can remain awake and aware. Or you may elect to continue life support measures even if you are sedated.

When symptoms are properly managed, death from lung cancer comes gently and peacefully. As tumors invade the lungs, energy diminishes and fatigue increases, reaching the point where it's difficult to get out of bed or stay awake for more than a brief period of time. Fluid may fill the lungs, causing coughing and difficulty breathing. Medication can prevent pain or breathlessness. Mental confusion may develop, but sedatives can soothe any agitation. Thirst and hunger disappear as the body shuts down. Breathing becomes shallow and irregular. In the final hours, intervals between breaths become longer. Then, at last, there are no more breaths and life is over.

Resources on Dying

The following resources provide both comfort and practical information. Some are available only online. If you don't have Internet access, ask a friend or a librarian to print them out for you.

entered a new phase, and she'd be dealing with it in a constructive way. I've spoken with many lung cancer patients and their families who have turned to hospice in the last weeks or months of illness. The overwhelming majority have felt that hospice greatly eased their final days.

I explained that hospice wouldn't change her medical treatment or her prognosis. Supportive care would keep her active and alert for as long as possible. At the same time, the hospice social worker and volunteers would help her work through the anger and fear she felt about dying. They would also review her financial arrangements and would facilitate discussions with her family, providing them with support too.

That was my last conversation with Joanne. She died about two months later. I was glad to hear that she entered an excellent hospice program three weeks before the end. I hope the staff helped her to die at peace.

Offering Support

Someone you care about is dying. What do you do? What do you say? People sometimes feel so overwhelmed by their emotions and so inadequate that they avoid talking about what is happening, and may even avoid visiting. A few suggestions:

- Offer to read aloud, talk, play music, pray, give a massage, hold hands, or simply sit silently.

- Admit that you don't know what to do and ask the patient for guidance.

- Don't be afraid to cry or to express your sadness.

- Listen, even if it's painful to hear what the dying person wants to say.

- Work on a project together, such as identifying family photographs or writing letters.

- If the patient is confused, respond in a neutral, loving way—for example: "I'm so sorry (or glad) to hear that," or "Tell me more." Keep conversation slow and simple. Identify yourself rather than asking, "Do you know who this is?"

- Always assume that you can be heard and understood, even if the patient is delirious or in a coma.

- *Home Care Guide for Advanced Cancer: When Quality of Life is the Primary Goal of Care*, an excellent free guide from the American College of Physicians, is available only online (*http://www.cancer.gov/cancerinfo/advancedcancer*).

- *Advanced Cancer: Living Each Day*, a helpful free booklet published by the National Cancer Institute, is available online (*http://www.cancer.gov*) or by calling 800-4-CANCER (800-422-6237).

- Cancer Care's online resources include an informative special section on end-of-life concerns (*http://www.cancercare.org/EndofLifeConcerns*).

- CancerBACUP, the leading cancer information service in the United Kingdom, has a fine booklet titled *Dying with Cancer*, which is available online (*http://www.cancerbacup.org.uk/info/dying.htm*).

- The Centering Corporation offers an extensive selection of books on death and grieving. See catalog online (*http://www.centering.org*) or call 402-553-1200.

We know that reading this chapter and thinking about the end of life will be painful. But we hope the information we've provided will also contribute to your peace of mind. Even when there is too little time, there is much you can accomplish for yourself and those you love. We wish you a meaningful and comforting journey.

AFTERWORD

You may have read this book because you or someone you love has been diagnosed with lung cancer. Or maybe you're concerned because you know you're at risk. We hope you found not only the information you were seeking, but also encouragement and hope. Lung cancer is a terrible disease. But today—thanks to the promise of early detection and to improved treatments—there's more reason for optimism than ever before.

Information and technology can win the war against lung cancer. But they're not enough. We need your help too. From the 1950s to the 1990s, the incidence of lung cancer increased by over 500 percent. In contrast, five-year survival rates barely budged, remaining under 15 percent to this day. The chief reason is that lung cancer usually isn't discovered until it has reached an advanced stage and causes symptoms. In addition, existing technology hasn't been used to its full potential to treat lung cancer. We desperately need more research, especially on early diagnosis. That can happen with your involvement.

In the 1980s we saw the emergence of another deadly disease: AIDS. Less than two decades later, AIDS mortality has plummeted. Like diabetes and heart disease, AIDS has become what lung cancer should be: a chronic illness that patients can expect to live with, not quickly die from. The rapid development of diagnostic tests and effective treatments for AIDS was not a matter of luck. AIDS patients and their loved ones mobilized and pressed for action, and money was poured into research.

Most of the limited public funding devoted to lung cancer treatment is focused on smoking cessation. Yes, that's very important. But more than half of those diagnosed with lung cancer are nonsmokers or people who've already quit. Even if cigarettes go the way of spittoons, lung cancer will remain at epidemic levels for many years. Breast cancer and colorectal cancer also are related to lifestyle choices, including lack of exercise and high-fat diets. Yet we don't devote nearly all our breast and colorectal cancer treatment dollars to prevention; considerable effort is given to diagnosis, therapies, and support for existing patients. Why not the same for those with lung cancer?

We hope so much that this book has helped you. We also hope it will inspire you to join the efforts of lung cancer advocates. Check the web sites of leading organizations—such as ALCASE (*http://www.alcase.org*) and Lung cancer.org (*http://www.lungcancer.org*)—to learn about current initiatives. Watch your local newspaper for announcements of Lung Cancer Awareness activities every November. Less than a century ago, lung cancer was a rare disease. With your involvement, we can begin to return it to the obscurity it deserves.

———

"There is a theory: we, humans, are merely a host for viruses. I remember being enchanted by that idea until I was diagnosed with lung cancer, then I wanted to turn the tables. I did not want to be a guest in my own body. I know our language for disease is poor: you do not fight these things, whatever 'these things' are: you learn to live with the fears and discomforts these things bring. We need less military language and more poetry to discuss cancer, AIDS, mental and emotional variations. We need a more humane way of looking, in fact, at life. Step by step we will not defeat cancer but we may lay it to rest quietly while we continue our life's journey."
    —Nikki Giovanni, poet and lung cancer survivor

GLOSSARY

We hope you will learn the vocabulary of lung cancer. You'll feel more in command if you understand what you read and what you hear from your medical team. This glossary lists terms that you're likely to encounter and provides brief definitions.

If the word you seek is not in this glossary, check the index or consult the following sources. And never hesitate to ask your doctor or oncology nurse to stop and explain what they're saying.

- *The Cancer Dictionary,* by Roberta Altman and Michael J. Sarg, M.D. *revised edition,* Checkmark Books, 1999)

- The National Cancer Institute's online dictionary (*http://www.cancer. gov/dictionary*)

———

Acupressure: An ancient Chinese medical technique in which pressure is exerted on particular points on the body that are believed to correspond to different organs.

Acupuncture: An ancient Chinese medical technique in which fine, flexible needles are inserted into particular points on the body that are believed to correspond to different organs.

Adenocarcinoma: The most common type of non-small cell lung cancer.

Adjuvant chemotherapy: Chemotherapy that is given after surgery or radiation to kill any remaining cancer cells.

Adjuvant radiation therapy: Radiation therapy that is given after surgery to kill any remaining cancer cells.

Advance directives: Documents that allow individuals to guide decisions about their medical care even if they become incapacitated. See *living will* and *durable power of attorney for health care.*

Alopecia: Loss of hair on the head or on the body. Alopecia is a possible side effect of chemotherapy; radiation therapy can cause hair loss in the area through which the beam passes.

Alternative therapy: Healing approach that is not part of mainstream medical treatment and that is used instead of conventional treatment.

Alveoli: Clusters of microscopic sacs deep inside the lungs where oxygen and carbon dioxide are transferred to and from the bloodstream.

Americans with Disabilities Act (ADA): A law that prohibits some forms of discrimination against people with disabilities, including cancer.

Analgesic: Painkiller.

Anemia: A condition in which the bone marrow does not produce sufficient red blood cells. Symptoms include fatigue and shortness of breath. Chemotherapy and radiation can cause anemia.

Angiogenesis: Development of blood vessels. As a cancerous tumor develops, angiogenesis supports its growth. See *anti-angiogenesis drugs.*

Anti-angiogenesis drugs: A therapeutic approach to cancer that attempts to starve tumors by cutting off their blood supply. See *angiogenesis.*

Apoptosis: Genetic instructions that cause cells to destroy themselves if they become infected or damaged. Also called programmed cell death.

Arterial blood gas analysis (ABG): Measurement of oxygen, carbon dioxide, and other gases in a sample of blood drawn from an artery. The purpose is to assess lung performance.

Artery: Blood vessel that carries blood away from the heart.

Asbestos: A mineral, previously used in construction and manufacturing, that breaks into tiny fibers when crushed. If inhaled, the fibers may cause lung cancer. See *malignant mesothelioma.*

Auscultation: Listening by a doctor during a medical checkup. By listening to breathing sounds with a stethoscope pressed to an individual's chest or upper back, a doctor can check the respiratory system for fluid or other obstructions.

Belly breathing: Breathing by using the bellows-like power of the diaphragm, the muscle under the lungs, to maximize the exchange of air with each breath. Also called abdominal or diaphragmatic breathing.

Benign: Abnormal growth that is not cancerous, though it may be harmful in other ways. See *malignant.*

Beta-carotene: A form of vitamin A, found in yellow and orange vegetables and fruits, which may play a role in lung cancer prevention.

Bi-lobectomy: Surgical removal of two out of the three lobes of a right lung.

Biopsy: Extraction of a small sample of tissue or fluid for examination under a microscope.

Blood-brain barrier: Special blood vessels that prevent most chemicals from entering the brain.

Blood count: Test performed on a blood sample to determine if an individual has normal quantities of white blood cells, red blood cells, and platelets.

Board-certified doctor: A doctor who has undergone at least three years of specialized training in addition to medical school, and who has met certification standards of an organization recognized by the American Board of Medical Specialties and the American Medical Association.

Bone marrow: Tissue inside bones that produces blood cells.

Brachytherapy: A form of radiation therapy in which a small amount of radioactive material is placed inside the body, near or in a tumor or in the area from which a tumor has been removed.

Breakthrough pain: Episodes of pain that occur despite use of painkillers.

Breastbone: The long flat bone that runs down the center of the chest, to which the ribs are attached. Also called sternum.

Bronchi: See *bronchus.*

Bronchiole: One of the smaller airways that branch from the bronchi.

Bronchoalveolar carcinoma (BAC): A form of non-small cell lung cancer that causes mucus-producing cells to proliferate on the walls of the alveoli.

Bronchoscope: A long, flexible telescope, equipped with fiber-optic light and a camera, that is used to examine the bronchi.

Bronchoscopy: Examination of the bronchi with a bronchoscope.

Bronchus: One of two large airways that conduct air in and out of the two lungs. Plural: *bronchi.*

Bupropion: A prescription drug, used as an antidepressant (Wellbutrin) and also sold in smaller doses as Zyban, to counter the effects of nicotine withdrawal.

Cachexia: A disabling condition characterized by muscle wasting, loss of appetite, and weight loss. Can occur as the result of cancer.

Cancer: Uncontrolled growth of abnormal cells that invades adjacent tissue and spreads to new sites in the body.

Carcinogen: Cancer-causing chemical, radiation, or virus.

Carcinogenesis: The process of cancer development.

Catheter: A tube installed in the body, permanently or temporarily, through which fluids can be drained or administered.

CAT scan: See *CT scan.*

Cell: Fundamental unit of living organisms.

Chemoprevention: Medication, including vitamin or mineral supplements, intended to prevent cancer.

Chemotherapy: Treatment of cancer with drugs that interfere with the metabolism and replication of cells.

Chromosome: In humans, one of twenty-three pairs of DNA strands that carry genes and transmit hereditary information. See *DNA.*

Chronic bronchitis: A condition, usually smoking-related, in which the airways become chronically irritated and infected, producing coughing, shortness of breath, and fatigue.

Chronic obstructive pulmonary disease (COPD): A condition in which a person suffers from both chronic bronchitis and emphysema.

Cilia: Microscopic hair-like projections that grow from the walls of the airways. The cilia sweep particles, germs, and other debris out of the respiratory system.

Clinical research: A study conducted by health care professionals involving people rather than animals, microorganisms, or cells.

Clinical trials: A series of studies designed to determine if treatment measures are both effective and reasonably safe for humans.

Cobalt-60: A radioactive version of cobalt that emits gamma rays and is sometimes used as a radiation source in radiation therapy.

COBRA: See *Consolidated Omnibus Reconciliation Act.*

Combination chemotherapy: See *concurrent chemotherapy.*

Combined modality treatment: Treatment of cancer with a combination of two or three approaches, including surgery, chemotherapy, and radiation. Sometimes called combined treatment.

Comfort care: See *palliative care.*

Compassionate use: An FDA-sanctioned procedure that allows individual patients to receive experimental drugs outside of clinical trials. Also called emergency use or single-patient IND (Investigational New Drug). This term is sometimes used to describe the patient assistance programs through which drug companies provide medication for patients who can't afford to pay for it.

Complementary and alternative medicine (CAM): A very wide range of healing approaches that have not traditionally been part of conventional medical treatment in the United States.

Complementary therapy: Healing approach that has not traditionally been part of mainstream medical treatment and that is used in addition to conventional treatment.

Complete lymph node dissection: In lung cancer treatment, removal of all the lymph nodes in the mediastinum.

Complete remission: A response to cancer treatment in which all evidence of cancer disappears.

Concurrent chemotherapy: Chemotherapy given at the same time as radiation therapy. Also called combination chemotherapy.

Consolidated Omnibus Reconciliation Act (COBRA): A law that allows former employees and their spouses to temporarily keep group health insurance obtained from an employer.

Consolidation chemotherapy: A second round of chemotherapy administered after an initial round. The purpose is to kill any remaining cancer cells.

Contralateral: Pertaining to the opposite side.

Cranial irradiation: Radiation of the entire brain for the treatment or prevention of cancerous brain tumors or metastases. See *prophylactic cranial irradiation.*

CT scan: Also called CAT scan (computed axial tomography). A diagnostic test that uses a series of x-rays and computers to create internal views of the body.

Cytology: Study of cells.

Diaphragm: A flat muscle separating the upper and lower parts of the torso, whose up and down motion moves air in and out of the lungs.

Differentiation: The process by which cells acquire specialized capabilities and characteristic appearance as they divide.

Digital clubbing: Changes in the fingers that are associated with lung and heart disease. Alterations include widening of the fingertips and an increase in the curve of the nails from cuticle to tip.

DNA (deoxyribonucleic acid): The chemical of which genes are made.

"Do not resuscitate" order (DNR): A document that individuals can use to inform medical personnel that they do not wish medical intervention if their heartbeat or breathing stops.

Dose limiting: A side effect of chemotherapy that can limit the dose or frequency of future treatments.

Dosimetrist: A technician who calculates the time each radiation treatment should last to deliver the dose prescribed by the radiation oncologist.

Double-blind study: Clinical research in which neither the investigators nor the patients know who is getting which treatment.

Doubling time: The time it takes for cells to divide, thereby doubling in number.

Durable power of attorney for health care: A legal document in which individuals can name a trusted person to make medical decisions on their behalf if they become incapacitated.

Dysphagia: Difficulty swallowing.

Dysplasia: Abnormal, premalignant cells that don't look or function like their normal counterparts. Dysplasia occurs early in the development of cancer.

Dyspnea: Uncomfortable shortness of breath.

Edema: Swelling of the body or part of the body, such as the ankles, which is caused by fluid retention.

Emesis: Vomiting.

Emphysema: A condition that is usually smoking-related in which the walls between the alveoli break down, making them less efficient at transferring oxygen and carbon dioxide to and from the bloodstream. A common symptom of emphysema is shortness of breath.

Esophagitis: Inflammation of the esophagus. A common side effect when radiation is given to the center of the chest.

Esophagus: The tube that connects the throat to the stomach.

False negative: An incorrect test result indicating that an existing condition is not present.

False positive: An incorrect test result indicating that a condition is present when it is not.

Family and Medical Leave Act (FMLA): A law that requires some employers to permit workers to take unpaid leave for their own or a family member's medical treatment.

FDA: See *Food and Drug Administration.*

FEV$_1$ (forced expiratory volume in one second): The amount of air that can be expelled from the lungs in one second, as measured by spirometry.

Fibrosis: Formation of fibrous tissue. Can occur as the result of disease or of treatment.

Fine needle aspiration: Technique for obtaining a biopsy in which a very thin hollow needle is inserted into the body and into a suspect area, using an x-ray or CT scan for guidance.

Fluorescent bronchoscopy: A diagnostic procedure in which bronchoscopy is performed under the illumination of a special kind of fluorescent light. See *bronchoscopy.*

Food and Drug Administration (FDA): Governmental agency that regulates the sale of drugs and other medical treatments and is responsible for reviewing and monitoring research findings on their safety and efficacy.

Fractions: In radiation therapy, the amount of the total radiation dose administered in each treatment session.

Frozen section: A very thin slice of tissue that has been quick-frozen and then cut for immediate examination under a microscope. In cancer treatment, used during surgery when a tissue sample has been obtained to provide rapid confirmation that cancer is present.

FVC (forced vital capacity): Total volume of air that can be expelled from the lungs in one full exhalation, as measured by spirometry.

Gamma rays: A type of radiation that is used for radiation therapy. See *cobalt-60.*

Gene: The basic unit of heredity, which directs development of a particular characteristic in an individual.

Genome: The set of approximately 30,000 genes that provide complete instructions for an individual's development.

Giant cell carcinoma: A form of non-small cell lung cancer.

Grade: In cancer diagnosis, an evaluation of tumor cells to determine how differentiated they are. The less differentiated, the more abnormal the cells and the more aggressive the cancer is likely to be.

Growth factor: A protein that promotes cell growth. Growth factor treatments that boost blood cell production are used to counter myelosuppression during cancer treatment. Other growth factors may play a role in the development of cancer; growth factor inhibitors are under investigation as cancer treatments.

Hemoptysis: Coughing up blood from the respiratory tract.

Health Insurance Portability and Accountability Act (HIPAA): A law offering limited protections to people who already have health insurance but are threatened with the loss of benefits.

HER/2neu: An oncogene that has been linked to lung cancer.

Hilum: In the respiratory system, the point at which a bronchus and associated blood vessels and nerves enter a lung.

Hospice: An approach to end-of-life care that emphasizes physical and emotional comfort, rather than curative treatment.

Hyperfractionated: A schedule for radiation therapy in which the total dose is divided into very small fractions, with treatments given more than once a day.

Hyperplasia: Excess cell growth that occurs early in cancer development.

Immune system: The many mechanisms that defend the body against infection and disease, including cancer.

Induction chemotherapy: Chemotherapy given as the first treatment for cancer.

Inflammation: Swelling and redness of tissues in response to irritation or infection.

Informed consent: Process by which investigators disclose all the risks and benefits to a patient who is about to undergo treatment or participate in clinical research.

Infusion: In medicine, administration of fluids or medications into the bloodstream through a vein.

Inspiratory muscle trainer: A device used to exercise and strengthen the muscles involved in respiration.

Institutional Review Board (IRB): A group at a hospital, university, or other research site that reviews proposed studies to make sure participants won't be exposed to inappropriate risks.

Integrative medicine: A term used by mainstream cancer centers and teaching hospitals for a healing approach that integrates complementary therapies with conventional treatments.

Intravenous: Administered through a vein.

Ipsilateral: Pertaining to the same side.

Large cell carcinoma: A form of non-small cell lung cancer.

Laser: A device that concentrates light into an intense, narrow beam that can cut or destroy tissue.

Lesion: An abnormal area in an organ or tissue.

Leukocytes: White blood cells that attack germs and other threats to the body, including precancerous cells.

Leukopenia: Insufficiency of white blood cells, which decreases a person's ability to fight infection, disease, and injury.

Limited resection: In lung cancer treatment, surgical removal of only the cancerous portion of a lobe and nearby tissue.

Linear accelerator: A machine used to produce x-rays for radiation therapy.

Living will: A document in which an individual specifies preferred treatment choices at the end of life.

Lobe: Section of the lungs. A normal right lung has three lobes; the left lung has two.

Lobectomy: Surgical removal of a lobe of a lung.

Lymph: A fluid containing white blood cells that bathes the tissues of the body, including the lungs, helping to fight infections.

Lymphatic vessels: A network of thin tubes that carry lymph throughout the body.

Lymph node: One of many small organs along the lymphatic vessels that filter lymph to remove bacteria and other material that might damage the body.

Magnetic resonance imaging: See *MRI.*

Malignant: Abnormal growth that is cancerous, capable of invading surrounding tissues and spreading to other parts of the body. See *benign.*

Malignant mesothelioma: A rare cancer, often caused by asbestos, that affects the mesothelial cells, which are found in the lining of the stomach and in the pleura.

Malignant pleural effusion: Fluid in the space between the lungs and the chest wall that contains malignant cells.

Mediastinoscopy: A procedure in which a viewing instrument and sometimes other instruments are inserted into the front of the chest to view the mediastinum and possibly collect tissue samples.

Mediastinum: Space between the two lungs.

Medical oncologist: A doctor who specializes in treating cancer with chemotherapy.

Metastasis: Process by which cancer cells migrate (or metastasize) from the original tumor to other parts of the body via the bloodstream or the lymphatic system. These distant cancers are called metastases or secondary tumors.

MRI (magnetic resonance imaging): A diagnostic test that uses a magnetic field to create images of the inside of the body.

Multi-modality treatment: See *combined modality treatment.*

Myc: An oncogene that has been linked to lung cancer.

Myelosuppression: Reduced bone marrow activity that results in fewer white blood cells, red blood cells, or platelets.

National Cancer Institute (NCI): Governmental agency within the National Institutes of Health that is concerned with many aspects of cancer research and education.

Neoadjuvant chemotherapy: Chemotherapy given prior to cancer treatment by surgery or radiation.

Neoadjuvant radiation therapy: Radiation therapy given prior to cancer treatment by surgery.

Neuropathy: Malfunction of the nerves that can be a side effect of chemotherapy. Symptoms include numbness, weakness, and pain.

Neutropenia: A condition in which the body has insufficient neutrophils and immune function is impaired.

Neutrophil: A type of white blood cell that specializes in fighting germs.

New primary: In a cancer survivor, a subsequent cancer that is not a metastasis of a previous cancer and that appears to have developed independently. Can be of the same type as earlier cancer or of a different type.

Nicotine: The addictive component of cigarettes.

Nocebo effect: A negative health effect produced by the power of suggestion. Opposite of *placebo.*

Nodule: Small, solid mass.

Non-small cell lung cancer (NSCLC): One of the two main categories of lung cancer. Includes adenocarcinoma, bronchoalveolar carcinoma (BAC), squamous carcinoma, large cell carcinoma, and giant cell carcinoma.

Nonsteroidal anti-inflammatory drug (NSAID): A category of painkillers for low-to-moderate-intensity pain that includes aspirin, ibuprofen, and naproxen sodium.

Oat cell carcinoma: See *small cell lung cancer.*

Off-label treatment: Use of an FDA-approved drug or other treatment for a purpose other than that for which it has specific approval.

Oncogenes: Genes that promote cell growth and multiplication, but that do not respond to signals that normally control cell proliferation. The result can be cancerous growth. See *proto-oncogene.*

Oncologist: A doctor who specializes in treating cancer.

Oncology: Study of the development, diagnosis, treatment, and prevention of cancer.

Oncology nurse (OCN or AOCN): A registered nurse who has received additional training in the care of cancer patients.

Opioid: Narcotic painkiller that can relieve severe pain, including morphine, codeine, fentanyl, and oxycodone.

Pack-year: A measure of exposure to tobacco carcinogens, defined as the equivalent of smoking one pack of cigarettes per day for a year.

Palliative care: Treatment that is aimed at prolonging life and maintaining the best possible quality of life rather than at curing disease. Also called comfort care.

Palpate: To examine by touching.

Paraneoplastic syndromes: Symptoms caused by hormones or other substances that are secreted by cancer tumors.

Partial remission: A response to cancer treatment in which the cancerous area is reduced but does not disappear.

Pathologist: A doctor who specializes in diagnosis of disease through tissue examination and laboratory tests.

Patient-controlled analgesia (PCA): Delivery of pain medication intravenously in very small doses via a pump that the patient controls.

Peripheral neuropathy: Tingling, pain, or loss of sensation in the feet or hands.

p53: A gene that normally senses genetic abnormalities and triggers apoptosis (programmed cell death). Abnormal p53 genes are found in most lung cancer cells.

Photodynamic therapy (PDT): In lung cancer treatment, a bronchoscopic procedure in which a patient is injected with a photosensitizing drug and an airway tumor is targeted with a red laser light.

Placebo: A look-alike treatment that actually contains no active ingredients. Used in some clinical trials (but only rarely in cancer trials) as a baseline to which active treatment is compared.

Platelet: Blood cell that helps control bleeding by causing clotting. Also called thrombocyte.

Pleura: A slippery membrane that covers the lobes of the lungs and the inside of the chest cavity, allowing the lungs to move smoothly during breathing.

Pleural effusion: A condition in which fluid accumulates in the space between the lungs and the pleura.

Pneumonectomy: Surgical removal of an entire lung.

Pneumonia: Infection of the lungs.

Port: In chemotherapy, a device implanted under the skin that allows drugs to be administered directly into a large vein inside the chest.

Positron emission tomography (PET): An imaging test that highlights areas where sugar metabolism is particularly rapid, possibly signaling cancer. In lung cancer, used during diagnosis to detect metastases and to assess the effectiveness of treatment.

Prognosis: Prediction about the course and outcome of a disease, based on experience with many patients.

Programmed cell death: See *apoptosis.*

Prophylactic cranial irradiation (PCI): Radiation treatment for the entire brain, sometimes given to lung cancer patients to prevent brain metastases.

Prostate, lung, colorectal, and ovarian cancer screening trial (PLCO): A National Cancer Institute screening study intended to learn if certain tests could reduce deaths from prostate, lung, colorectal, or ovarian cancer.

Protocol: In medicine, a plan that details the treatments a patient will receive.

Proto-oncogenes: Genes that instruct cells to divide. Proto-oncogenes can mutate or become defective and turn into cancer-causing oncogenes. See *oncogenes.*

Protraction: In radiation therapy, the length of time over which radiation is given.

Pulmonary: Relating to the lungs.

Pulmonary embolism: A life-threatening medical condition in which a clot blocks a major blood vessel in the lungs.

Pulmonary hypertension: A condition in which blood pressure is elevated in the blood vessels of the lungs.

Pulmonologist: A doctor who specializes in treating disorders of the chest.

Pulse oximetry: A test that measures how much oxygen the blood contains, performed by attaching a sensor to a finger, toe, or earlobe.

Pursed-lip breathing: Exhaling through pursed lips, as a way to exercise the muscles used to exhale or as a means of relieving stress.

Quality of life: General ability of a person to enjoy and participate in activities of normal life.

Radiation fibrosis: Scarring of lung tissue as a result of radiation therapy.

Radiation necrosis: Accumulated dead tissue from a tumor treated by radiation therapy.

Radiation oncologist: A doctor who specializes in treating cancer with radiation therapy.

Radiation physicist: A professional with training and expertise in the equipment used to deliver radiation therapy.

Radiation pneumonitis: Inflammation of healthy lung tissue as a result of radiation therapy.

Radiation port or **radiation portal:** The skin through which the rays pass during radiation therapy.

Radiation protectors: Experimental drugs that shield normal cells from damage during radiation therapy.

Radiation recall: Abnormal skin sensitivity in an area treated with radiation therapy in an individual previously treated with chemotherapy. Or similar sensitivity that emerges during chemotherapy in an individual who was treated earlier with radiation therapy.

Radiation sensitizers: Experimental drugs that make cancer cells more sensitive to the damaging effects of radiation.

Radiation technologist: A technician who positions patients during radiation therapy and administers treatment.

Radiation therapy: Use of rays to damage or kill cancer cells. Also called radiotherapy.

Radioactive antibodies: Experimental treatment in which radioactive antibodies are injected into the body. The antibodies seek out tumors and the radiation destroys them. This approach is called radioimmunotherapy.

Radioimmunotherapy: See *radioactive antibodies.*

Radiologist: A doctor who specializes in the diagnosis of cancer and other diseases with the use of radiation.

Radiosurgery: A form of radiation therapy that involves one to three high doses of radiation. Used in lung cancer mostly to treat small brain metastases.

Radiotherapy: See *radiation therapy.*

Radon: A colorless, odorless radioactive gas that is found in soil. Can cause lung cancer if inhaled over long periods of time.

Randomized clinical trial: Research in which participants are divided by chance into groups that receive different treatments, allowing the outcomes to be compared.

Ras: An oncogene that has been linked to lung cancer.

Recurrent cancer: Cancer that has returned after treatment.

Remission: After treatment by chemotherapy or radiation, evidence of cancer has disappeared (complete remission) or has been reduced (partial remission).

Rescue medication: Supplemental medication used for symptoms, such as breakthrough pain, that occur despite other treatment.

Resect: Surgically remove.

Resectable: Able to be removed surgically.

Respiratory system: The system of the body involved in breathing, including the nose, throat, larynx, trachea, bronchi, and lungs.

Retinoids: Derivatives of vitamin A that are essential for normal cell differentiation and that may be valuable for chemoprevention.

Risk factor: Any factor that increases a person's risk for a particular condition.

Screening: Checking for the presence of disease in people who appear to be healthy.

Secondary tumors: See *metastasis.*

Secondhand smoke: A mix of smoke exhaled by smokers (mainstream smoke) and smoke from burning tobacco (sidestream smoke) that contains the same carcinogens as the smoke inhaled by smokers.

Selenium: An essential trace mineral that appears to have chemopreventive potential for lung cancer.

Sentinel node: The first lymph node into which a tumor drains.

Sentinel node sampling: A procedure in which a tumor is injected with dye so that the movement of lymph can be tracked and the sentinel node identified.

Side effect: An unintended effect of treatment, usually unwanted.

Simulation: In radiation therapy, a preliminary session in which the radiation oncologist maps the area to be treated, using a beam of laser light instead of radiation.

Single-blind study: Clinical research in which patients don't know which treatment they are receiving, but the doctors do.

Single-patient IND: See *compassionate use*.

Sleeve resection: Surgical removal of a section of an airway and nearby lung tissue, but not an entire lobe.

Small cell lung cancer (SCLC): One of the two main categories of lung cancer. Sometimes called oat cell carcinoma, because the cells resemble oats under the microscope.

Spirometer: A device that measures the volume and speed of air movement in order to assess pulmonary function. See *FVC* and *FEV₁*.

Spirometry: Measurement of pulmonary function with a spirometer.

Sputum: Coughed-up material from the respiratory tract.

Sputum cytology: Microscopic examination of sputum. Used to detect cancerous cells shed from the lungs and airways.

Squamous carcinoma: A form of non-small cell lung cancer.

Staging: A standardized way of classifying cancer according to how advanced it is.

Stenosis: Narrowing or constriction of a passageway, such as an airway or a blood vessel.

Stent: A short tube that is implanted into a constricted airway or blood vessel to hold it open.

Stereotactic radiosurgery: A high-dose version of three-dimensional conformal radiotherapy that usually involves just one to three treatments. Systems include Gamma Knife, X-Knife, CyberKnife, and Peacock.

Sternum: See *breastbone*.

Superior vena cava: Vein that runs through the mediastinum.

Superior vena cava syndrome: Symptoms—including swelling of the face and upper body, distended veins in the neck, and rapid breathing—caused by a tumor blocking the superior vena cava.

Supportive care: In cancer treatment, measures that help counter symptoms or side effects.

Surgical oncologist: A doctor who specializes in performing surgery to treat cancer.

Synergistic: Characteristic of interacting forces, where the combined effect is multiplied rather than added.

Symptom: An abnormality of the body or its functions.

Telomere: Section at the end of each chromosome thread, a piece of which disappears each time a cell divides. When the telomere is gone, the cell dies.

Terminal: An advanced stage of disease in which life expectancy is limited.

Terminal sedation: Use of narcotic painkillers and sedatives, plus withdrawal of artificial feeding and intravenous fluids, to promote comfort at the end of life without concern for shortening life.

Thoracentesis: A procedure in which pleural effusion is drained or extracted to relieve symptoms or to check for the presence of cancerous cells.

Thoracic: Referring to the thorax.

Thoracic surgeon: A doctor who is specially trained to perform surgery involving the chest cavity.

Thoracoscope: An instrument used to view the inside of the chest.

Thoracoscopy: A procedure in which a thoracoscope and possibly other instruments are inserted into the chest to view the lining of the chest and the surface of the lungs, and possibly collect tissue samples.

Thoracotomy: Any surgical operation that enters the chest.

Thorax: The chest—the upper half of the body, between the neck and the diaphragm.

Three-dimensional conformal radiation therapy: A form of radiation therapy that uses advanced imaging technology and computer simulation to map the location, shape, and dimensions of a cancerous tumor so that beams can be directed from multiple angles to converge on the tumor.

Thrombocyte: See *platelet*.

Thrombocytopenia: Insufficient platelets, the component of blood that enables it to clot.

Tissue margin: A border of healthy tissue surrounding cancerous tissue that has been surgically removed or treated by radiation therapy.

Trachea: The tube between the larynx and the bronchi. Also called windpipe.

Transcutaneous Electric Nerve Stimulation (TENS): A method of blocking pain by applying mild electric currents to the skin.

Treatment-naive: A person with cancer who has not yet been treated with chemotherapy or radiation therapy. An individual who has been treated with surgery is sometimes (but not always) considered treatment-naive.

Tumor: A mass of abnormal tissue, which may be benign or malignant.

Tumor board: A team of specialists who review the records and test results of cancer patients and then make treatment recommendations.

Tumor-suppressor genes: Genes that halt cell division.

Vein: Blood vessel that carries blood to the heart.

Video-assisted thoracic surgery (VATS): Procedure in which thoracic surgery is performed through small incisions between ribs using special viewing and operating instruments.

Visceral pleura: Part of the pleural membrane that surrounds and separates the lobes of the lungs.

X-ray: A form of radiation that is used in low doses to diagnose disease and in high doses to treat cancer.

Index

Page numbers in *italics* refer to illustrations.

ABOUT THE AUTHORS

Claudia I. Henschke, Ph.D., M.D., is Chief, Division of Chest Imaging, at the New York Presbyterian Hospital–Cornell Medical Center and Professor of Radiology, Department of Radiology, at the Weill Medical College of Cornell University.

For the past decade, Dr. Henschke's research has focused on early diagnosis of lung cancer. She is author or coauthor of more than two hundred research papers published in distinguished peer-reviewed journals. Dr. Henschke has served on national committees that review grant applications and set policy and professional standards, including committees of the Agency for Health Care Policy, the National Institutes of Health, the National Academy of Science, the Radiological Society of North America, and the American College of Radiology.

Peggy McCarthy, MBA, founder and president of McCarthy Medical Marketing, Inc., and Innovative Medical Education Consortium, Inc., is a nationally recognized cancer patient advocate. She is founder of ALCASE (The Alliance for Lung Cancer Advocacy, Support, and Education), and a founding member and secretary of the Board of Directors of ACORE (Association for Communication in Oncology through Research and Education). She serves on the National Dialogue on Cancer and the American College of Chest Physicians Task Force on Women, Smoking and Lung Cancer, as well as on several committees and boards of the National Cancer Institute. In 2000, *Ladies' Home Journal* recognized her contributions by naming her as one of the year's "women to watch" in women's medicine.

Sarah Wernick, Ph.D., is an award-winning freelance health writer. Her books include the best-selling *Strong Women Stay Young* (Bantam, 1997 and 2000). In 1997 she received the American Medical Association President's Prize for excellence in tobacco reporting for "The Silent Killer," published in *Ladies' Home Journal*—the first feature article about lung cancer to appear in a major woman's magazine.

Visit the web site for *Lung Cancer: Myths, Facts, Choices—and Hope*
http://www.lungcancerhope.com